Mama Bear

Mama Bear

One Black Mother's Fight for Her Child's Life and Her Own

Shirley Smith

with Zelda Lockhart

HARPER

An Imprint of HarperCollins*Publishers*

HarperCollins books may be purchased for educational, business, or sales promotional use. For information, please email the Special Markets Department at SPsales@harpercollins.com.

FIRST EDITION

Designed by Leah Carlson-Stanisic

Library of Congress Cataloging-in-Publication Data has been applied for.

ISBN 978-0-06-301078-9

21 22 23 24 25   LSC   10 9 8 7 6 5 4 3 2 1

This book is dedicated to my mother, Bertina Marie Harris. Without your life I wouldn't have a story to tell. You are forever in my heart. Thank you for your life. Thank you for your struggle. Thank you for your strength and thank you for your transparency. And of course to my three D's, my cubs, my beautiful virtuous daughters—Demi, Dakota, and Denver. As long as God gives me breath, I will do my best to show you the best version of myself and be an image that you will be proud to look up to.

Contents

Contents

Contents

Introduction

This book was brewing in me since my days of being eight years old and hiding in the closet writing in my little diary. But it was a cold Sunday, in February 2018, a little more than a year after I'd given birth to Dakota and she'd survived 141 days in the NICU, that solidified the call for me to write my story. My ten-year-old Demi, my one-year-old Dakota, and I were away from our faith community in New Jersey, the Love of Jesus Family Church. We were in Ohio for JR's season on the road with the Cavaliers. I was pregnant with our next child, Denver, overwhelmed with postpartum blues, pregnancy blues, mama-of-a-preteen blues. Needless to say, it was a time when I needed God's guidance.

On Saturday, the day before, I had a feeling and a push that said, *Get into the house,* meaning the church. I had a feeling to go to this different church, not one in Ohio I had tried visiting a few times. I was like, *Really God? An hour drive to church?* When I didn't receive a reply from God, I knew he wasn't playing. I felt the urge to invite my brother's girlfriend Jasmink to come with me. I thought to myself, *God you are on a roll ain't you? I don't even know if this girl goes to church.*

I did as instructed, and when I did, another weight was lifted. When I called Jasmink, she responded with joy, "I sure will. I need to go to church."

In the middle of the night that Saturday, I realized the devil was trying his best to keep me from making it out of the house to church the next morning. Dakota was off the hook the whole night. She was restless, congested, irritable, and I barely got any sleep. With JR on the road for work I had to cover the twenty-four-hour Dakota shift solo, alone.

Then, *buzz, buzz, buzz.* I was like, *I know that is not my alarm going off already. You've got to be kidding me.* Then I thought, *Eh, I can just go next week.* I battled with my thoughts for about thirty minutes before peeling myself out of bed. I felt like crap and looked like Beetlejuice. What pulled me through was how good God has been to me and my family during those months that things were touch-and-go with Dakota's life. I realized that the least I could do was go into "the house" and personally thank him. Besides, I was always taught that there is a blessing in your pressing. I got my pregnant self up, got Dakota dressed, told Demi to get ready, got Jasmink, and got on the road.

Introduction

All sorts of foolishness was going on as we drove to church. My Bluetooth connection was cutting on and off, so the gospel music we had planned for the hour drive was a no-go. It was freeze-raining, making the roads treacherous, and it was ten degrees. Then, we got lost.

We finally made it to the Burning Bush Church in Akron, Ohio, and skated inside to catch the tad bit of praise and worship that was still taking place. We were an hour late, but on time for what was next to come.

The minister talked about power moves and how it was time to breathe life into any dream you thought was dead. I will never forget how specifically he said, "It's time to write *that book*!"

All I could think was, *Wow God! This is why you were pressing me.*

All I could remember was standing there like a statue with Dakota on my hip, Demi at my side, and my new baby, Denver, in my womb. I was standing in the moment of grace and purpose after everything that I had been through. All I needed to do next was be obedient to God's plan.

This book is so important to me, because I want to help shed light on an issue that is foreign to many people. Black American women are twice as likely to lose their babies to preterm birth than their white counterparts—and almost four times as likely to experience maternal mortality. We have a 50 percent greater chance of dying in the period immediately following childbirth than our mothers before us. Basically, our children are endangered before being born.

Mama Bear

There are many factors that contribute to infant and maternal mortality that disproportionately affect Black American women, like early life traumas of physical abuse and neglect, and ongoing life stressors including experiencing extreme and moderate racism on a regular basis. Living with that kind of lifelong stress impacts Black American women's ability to fight off and recover from disease, and puts us and our infants at greater risk of losing our lives during the physical stress of childbearing and labor.

Living with childbirth as a health risk seems unthinkable in the age of modern medicine in America. But recent articles and studies have brought this issue of racial disparity in infant and maternal mortality rates to the public eye.

No one is immune: Both tennis champion Serena Williams and six-time Olympic track-and-field gold medalist Allyson Felix experienced life-threatening complications during childbirth despite their health-conscious lifestyles and professional and financial success. Beyoncé appeared on the cover of *Vogue* in September 2018 and detailed in its pages her experience with toxemia and the birth of her premature twins.

I am the wife of NBA Champion and All-Star JR Smith. I am yet another Black woman who despite doing everything right found myself stretched beyond endurance by the health complications of a severely preterm birth.

In this book, I offer the 141-day ordeal of fighting for my own life and that of my second daughter, Dakota, who is among the world's youngest preemies ever to survive. I parallel this

Introduction

journey with the story of my early life. Born into a childhood struggle to survive my mother's drug addiction, I had to take care of myself and my brother.

It is my story of loss, resilience, and the maternal instincts I gained over a lifetime that made all the difference when I entered the emergency room at the end of my twenty-first week of pregnancy on New Year's Day. I didn't bring my child home until May of that new year. The joys and pains of my life continue, but in the midst of it all, I hold to my belief in God, my family, and my love of journaling as the beacons to guide me in moments when I feel lost from myself.

I have written this book because it sheds light on the mind and body of someone who has lived the life that studies have concluded leads to maternal health issues and preterm birth. My story humanizes this Black-woman reality.

It is good to understand the whole journey of preterm birth so that we can look back and acknowledge the pain and make a promise to our bodies and to our children that we will heal and help them to see a brighter day. We can't help it that we had limited tools. We can't help it that our bodies held all of that multigenerational pain and disease. But we want our children's bodies to be the vessels of God's will. So we have to tell our complicated birth stories and tell the complicated life stories that led to that moment. Through sharing my story, I know I can lift someone up who is experiencing the same life challenges.

This book is more than the story of giving birth to one of the world's youngest preemies. I offer hope through the wisdom I gained by surviving childhood hardships. I offer my stories of looking for love, and eventually building love, with my husband, JR. I run the hope straight through the hardship to the day I thought all was wonderful in my life, where the difficulties of growing up with a mother on crack and an absent father seemed like they were behind me, only to have a stomachache in the middle of my pregnancy that turned out to be my daughter Dakota's birthday at only twenty-two weeks. I offer you the story of the Black superwoman breaking point. That breaking point was the moment that gave me the courage to look back at the building blocks of my life and heal, for myself and for my children. It was the point from which I gained the strength to start a nonprofit, My Kota Bear, that helps other families with preemies.

When I am doing my work with My Kota Bear, I am a vessel distributing the gifts and donations that folks have offered to other families of preemies, distributing the resources, the sense of community, the hope and resilience that I sometimes had and other times sorely needed.

This book is my way of continuing to be God's vessel. My story within the pages of this book is a shout-out to the power of maternal instincts, God, and therapeutic healing.

So yes, I offer the story of giving birth to one of the world's youngest preemies and being Black and the wife of an NBA All-Star who has to be on the road away from home all of the time. But while doing so, I let folks into my living room, welcome them into my home and to all of the things in my life that make me who I am. I want people to know how to create some self-care so they don't hit the wall of breakdown as hard as I did.

No shame. I have put it all out there in this book, but I don't leave people hanging. I share how I got through to this place where I have forgiven my mother and father for what they did and didn't do, forgiven myself and my body for what it could and couldn't do, and to this place where I am living a blessed life with my daughters and am able to help others do the same.

With this book, I take the miracle of my and Dakota's survival and use it as a tool to help other women understand how our bodies struggle to bring a new life into this world. I want families to know that they are not alone and that we can help each other raise our children.

PART I

Maternal Instincts When Nothing Else Makes Sense

A body doesn't just randomly break down and struggle with childbirth the way that mine did. We go through things as Black girls where we are born into the same hardships that our mothers were born into. The body holds on to all of that pain of the racism that it experiences every day, of the shame of poverty and not having what you need, of the secrets because some male family member or some boy at school touched you the wrong way. The body holds the time you were left alone because your parents didn't know any better or were caught up in their own storm of survival. And we have to root about to reconnect our instincts by writing in our journals, connecting with God, staying tight with our communities, and making new bonus family where we can.

Some maternal instincts are just there on the ready when you give birth; you are just born with them and they kick into action when it's time. Other maternal "knowhow"? Well, you just have to find your way back to that, because childhood trauma can block instincts or mess with the body's stress levels so much that you don't know up from down.

Dakota's birth taught me that when my own maternal instincts don't kick in, I can't go around confused and in pain until one of God's helpers shows up. Sometimes, I have to holler for help, holler like I ain't never hollered, in order to do my part in making sure one of God's helpers can show up and help me push the reset button on how to nurture myself and my children.

1

Kota Bear

You can never take for granted those times in life where you get a little peace in the middle of the storm. Those times when everything is great. It's like the body gets calm and feels safe and it knows that it is okay to get real. And then, everything that's been holed up in your body for so long feels comfortable enough in all that peace to unleash.

Broadview Heights, Ohio, December 31, 2016
It was New Year's Eve, and everything was sweet. Lauryn Hill was playing through the Bluetooth speakers. My mother-in-law, Ma, moved around me. She was my elder, and the queen in my kitchen. She gently coaxed, "Shirley, stir the greens. Stir the black-eyed peas, Shirley." Stir this, stir that.

"Yes ma'am."

We moved like yin and yang, humming one tune or another. The things we didn't need to talk about put us on the same accord: we both loved to cook and entertain family and we both lost our mothers at a young age. That song came on: "That thing, that thing, that thing." I did Lauryn's rap. Ma did the beatbox. She cracked me up when she just about spit out the black-eyed peas she was tasting to get down in the beat. Her shoulders all hunched up.

I had on my makeup and earrings but never managed to change out of my blue satin bathrobe or my headscarf, and that was okay because everybody in the house was family. My father-in-law, Pop; JR; and JR's friend Big Nick were in the den watching the game. JR's brothers, Chris and Dimitrius, were in the living room with our daughter Demi. JR and his brothers got their height from Pop, six foot seven, a muscular build, easily a 260-pound man. They were all tall, protective men, hanging out with Demi, who was curled up in her mermaid sleeping bag watching the Disney Channel and playing cards with her uncles, multitasking at eight years old like the best of them.

I rubbed my little baby bump so Dakota could get some of that love. I had seen our Dakota in the sonogram. She had JR's long forehead, and the shape of my high cheekbones. "Oh, yeah. Oh, yeah," I said to Ma when Lauryn got to singing "To Zion." I felt a chill go through my body, like Lauryn got it. She understood what it meant to come through a life of struggling to survive and put God and family first, to know that God is telling you everything is gonna be okay; even during those times when you have to eat the ashes of the earth to feed your family, everything is gonna be okay. Lord knows I had seen some troubled times, but God's grace held me in gratitude in that moment.

"A gift so great, is only one God could create." Ma sang along. Sing it! I held my hands on my Dakota under my robe. It was one of those moments where everything in the world feels like it's in the right place at the right time. One of those moments that I always wish I can hold still and cherish, because whenever it's like that, hell is just peeping around the corner.

The house was a blanket of humid mouthwatering smells: sweet cornbread that sat on the back of my tongue, onions, and Ma's secret ingredient of cumin in those black-eyed peas that woke up the sinuses. She liked to put a capful of vinegar in the greens that made you want to start chewing before the fork even got to your mouth. In my womb, Dakota was kicking like crazy to tell me to hurry up and eat.

We got in a circle and I said grace. We were about to see ourselves into a new year of new beginnings for our family. "Heavenly Father, bless this food, the friends and family around this circle, and the new life that is growing in me."

"Amen," and everybody got their plates and settled in either at the counter, the TV, or the dining room table. I took my plate to the counter with Ma and Pop and ate good listening to whatever Ma was saying, "Yes ma'am," listening to Demi giggling at whatever was on TV.

7

After the meal, the grown folks sat down at the dining room table to play the card game Boo Ray. So much for all of that peace; we were about to get loud. Big Nick, who we call the class clown, dealt the cards. "Empty ya pockets, Big Nick is in the house!" He was only five foot eight but was a seriously big man. I was ready with my mouth half-open waiting for him to shut up, so I could come back at him and raise the laughter.

Suddenly pain ripped through me worse than any pain I'd ever felt, and I grabbed Big Nick's meaty arm. I tried not to puncture his skin but was holding on tight. Everybody stopped looking at their cards and turned to me all concerned. When the stabbing pain released, I let go of Big Nick and just laughed it off. "I'm just having some tummy trouble. I done ate too much, trying to keep up with Big Nick. Y'all come on, let's play."

Another pain hit me like a jolt of lightning. I just stopped moving for a minute. While everybody put up their bets, I pushed through it. I didn't want anybody worrying over a belly-ache. I felt nauseous, so it had to be a bellyache.

JR looked at me across the table with a slight pinch in his forehead. "You okay, babe?" I don't remember a New Year's Eve when I was able to have him home. It was a fluke that he broke his thumb and had to sit out the end of the season. He scratched his forehead with the cast on his right hand, trying to make sense of his cards before making a bet. He asked again without looking at me, "Ya good, babe?"

"Yeah, I'm good." I got up from the table and went in the

little guest bathroom. It hurt so bad, and that's the only thought I had time to have before I was there lifting the toilet lid and trying to keep my robe out of the way. I threw up everything I ate, black-eyed peas, greens, everything.

I went and sat down on the couch away from everybody at the table and watched TV with Demi, who was lying on the floor half-inside her mermaid fin. All those colors and the laughing box and high-pitched tones of whatever she was watching, and things went from sugar to shit in two point five seconds. My head was spinning, and I felt cold and hot like I was getting the flu or something.

JR peeped his head in the living room. "Babe, want me to play your hand?"

I could barely lift my head to say, "Honey, I'm gonna chill out and watch some TV."

They finished playing cards, we watched the ball drop, and I was struggling to be as normal as I could. Finally, everybody went to bed. Ma stayed downstairs doing the dishes and JR and I went upstairs. We were sitting up with the lights on trying to recap and laugh about the day, but those pains kept coming. I think I was mostly fooling myself, trying not to upset anybody—my whole life I had put myself second, always the one who kept it together for everyone else, never asking for help. But it seemed like JR, Ma, and Pop were on alert anyhow.

Pop yelled up to our bedroom in that deep James Earl Jones voice of his that made everybody listen. He kept it short, sweet, and to the point the way he always did. "Look, Shirley, if you aren't feeling better in the morning, I don't care that it is New Year's Day, I'm taking yo ass to the hospital."

I told him, "I think I'm fine. I just need to sleep."

JR asked, "Baby, don't you just want to go get it checked out?" I told him to go to sleep. He knew if I said I was okay, then there was no arguing with me. I reached over and turned off the light, telling myself I would be fine in the morning.

I couldn't rest all night. Every fifteen minutes the pain was so bad. Then, every ten minutes. I sat up in the dark and timed them on my phone and realized that just before sunrise they were five minutes apart, like labor pains—but that couldn't be! It was early New Year's morning, which put me at my last day of being twenty-one weeks pregnant.

I went to the bathroom, sat on the toilet, and put my cool hands on my tiny tummy. Dakota was sleeping in there like she should be. "Yeah everything is good." But then the next pain was so intense and a whole minute long, the pain traveling from my uterus all the way to my teeth. Denial is some powerful shit. We inherit that thing of denying our pain. So many of us are told growing up that showing our pain is a sign of weakness. So as Black women we just go around saying, "No, I'm not in pain. I'm okay. It's gonna be fine." And I can't tell you how many times that came out of my mouth during some of the most traumatic stuff I've ever been through. I had learned to deal with all levels of pain, emotional pain, physical pain, even labor pains y'all. As Black women we don't learn to say things like, *I'm in pain and I need this and that to happen.* Instead we worry about inconveniencing folks.

I stayed in the bathroom so I wouldn't disturb anybody with my grimacing, and then there was a little watery discharge. That's what broke my wall of denial. *God, what is happening? Please be okay, Dakota.*

I stood in the bathroom in my sweatpants and T-shirt, looking in the mirror, deciding what to do next without disturbing the whole house. Everybody was still asleep except JR's mother. I could hear her clanking around in the kitchen. I sat down on the edge of the bed, eased on a pair of sneakers, and held my voice calm. "JR, babe, I'm gonna have Ma run me to the hospital just to check it out."

He was half-asleep. "You okay?"

"It's just the pains, but it's nothing—probably a stomach bug."

Why do we do that? Why isn't it okay to hurt and to scream and holler so that someone will come to the rescue?

I kept my hand on my belly feeling for Dakota, and thanked God that she was stretching her feet against my hand. "I'm good, I'm good. I'll call you when I get there. Just go back to bed."

He agreed in his sleep. "Okay, babe."

I went to the top of the stairs and I could feel discharge trickle down my thigh. I reached in my sweatpants to touch it and saw it was clear, not bloody. I told myself, *It's not dripping down between your legs like it did when your water broke with Demi. It's just some discharge. This is not labor.*

"Come on, Dakota. Let's go check it out." I eased myself down the stairs toward Ma in the kitchen when another pain hit. I whisper-yelled from the stairs, "Ma! Can you please take me to the hospital?"

When I got to the bottom of the stairs, Ma was dressed but still had on a head rag and was swirling a pat of butter around in a pan. She looked up like she was seeing things. *"Shirley?"*

When she saw my sweatpants were wet, she dropped the frying pan. "I'm taking you to the hospital *right now.* You in labor, girl!" I sat down on the bottom stair. "No ma'am, that can't be, it's got to be something else." But she already had her coat on and mine in hand.

The hospital was thirty minutes away, but like a woman on a mission, Ma was flying through the streets of Broadview Heights and onto the highway to get to Cleveland Clinic's Hillcrest Hospital. I was curled into myself in the passenger seat, riding pains that were now about three minutes apart. My head was swimming and I had to keep my eyes closed; even the light of day made everything worse. I couldn't think, I couldn't breathe. Then I heard sirens and felt the car slowing down. I opened my eyes when Ma rolled her window down for a cop, who said, "Ma'am you know you're speeding." Then he saw me and said, "Oh, you are trying to get your daughter to the hospital . . ." Then he yelled, "Go, go, go!" and ran back to his car, and gave us an escort.

When we arrived at the hospital, Ma must have been nervous trying to deal with the situation and didn't think to pull in front of the emergency room door. After we parked, there was a bridge to cross to get to the entrance, and I just couldn't. A woman in scrubs saw us struggling and ran a wheelchair across the bridge. It took everything in me to just stay in that chair and not let the pain spill me out of it. That's when I knew for sure something was so wrong. I prayed, *God, please let Dakota be okay.*

I could see us getting closer to the doors and I concentrated on the red sign that said "emergency." Inside it was just a whirlwind of people asking my mother-in-law all of these questions and handling my body. I was in so much pain that the room was spinning, and parts of my body felt numb. They started asking me, "How long have you been in pain?" One minute I could talk, but the next minute, the pain would come and I couldn't say a word, so I couldn't explain it to them, but they kept asking questions anyway.

I finally managed to blurt out, "Where is my doctor?"

"She's on vacation."

There was a swarm of aqua scrubs and unfamiliar faces, and all of it was too much to register. Then this Black woman came over to me and her serene face stopped the swirl. She introduced herself calmly. "I am Dr. Diane Young."

I focused on her warm brown eyes as she said, "I'm here to see what's going on. I'm going to put these sensors on your stomach." So much was happening I didn't even realize that they had me in a bed, coat off, shoes off, lying on my back, wet sweatpants off, with a sheet draped over the bottom half of my body.

Unlike everybody else, Dr. Young told me each thing she was about to do before she did it. She was only about ten years older than me, but old enough for me to look at her broad, confident face and feel like I could finally breathe. She reminded me of my cousin Lynette. When I was twelve years old, Lynette— also only ten years older than me—was confident and strong enough to rescue me from our empty apartment and become my guardian.

Dr. Young had that kind of woman-take-control manner. I calmed down and let her put little pieces of tape and sensors on my belly. Her straight brown shoulder-length hair and dark-framed glasses gave her a look of authority. I told her, my voice all scratchy, "I'm just having pains and cramps in my stomach. Not labor pains, but something feels wrong."

Dr. Young stood there and read the printout with all the little Z's on it and said with her head tilted and her hand on my hand, "No, honey, these are contractions." She showed me how sharp and spiky the Z's were. "You're lucky your mother-in-law brought you in. These are definitely contractions."

I grew up one of those Black girls who knew how to get shit done, how to feed myself and my siblings if we were hungry, how to get somebody to come turn on the electricity when my mother didn't pay the bill. Dr. Young's words took my whole world and twisted it into something that I couldn't fix or control.

"*Excuse me?*" I just busted out crying. "No ma'am, that's not right." I started panicking. I was sweating. I was so confused. I knew a woman couldn't have a baby at just twenty-two weeks.

All of a sudden all of these nurses were coming in and out of the room. I called JR. I was boohooing through the phone. "Honey, please get here quick. Please get here. They said we are about to have Dakota now. She is about to come now."

He started yelling, *"What? What?"*

He and Pop must have sped; they got there in no time. When JR saw me, I was hooked up to all of this stuff. I could tell from looking in his eyes that he was trying to be strong and not burst out in tears. I had been given a safe dose of meds to calm the pain of the contractions, but that didn't mean I was ready for a big conversation. Everybody asked me questions as if I understood what was happening, rather than actually telling me what was happening to my body or to Dakota. I don't think they understood. I felt so exposed, like they knew something about me and my baby that I didn't, and no one would tell me what it was.

I didn't know what to do. This was very different from being forced to be a mother as a little girl and making decisions at eight years old. This wasn't being twenty-four and planning to have Demi, sitting around watching *A Baby Story* on TLC. Demi came right on time, without a worry, healthy. That was eight years ago. Here I was being fired at with questions I didn't know how to answer when I thought I knew what to expect with this pregnancy.

I still couldn't wrap my mind around this moment. How I went from eating New Year's dinner with my family, only a little more than halfway through my pregnancy, to lying in the hospital hooked up to machines. How can a baby be born this early? How could she survive that?

JR hadn't caught up with the reality yet either, and just kept stammering and smoothing his beard with his good hand. Between the intense pain, all the beeping noises, the smell of old peroxide, so many hands and new people and their damned questions, I just lost it. I yelled, "No one is going to touch my body! Get off my damned body! Somebody needs to tell me what is happening!"

Dr. Young cleared the room, pulled up a chair, and held my hand. "Honey, let me explain to you and your husband what's going on. It's looking like you are going to have your daughter as a premature birth. She is going to come soon, but we are going to give you a dose of medication that will stop your contractions. We'll elevate your bottom to try to keep her up there for as many days or hours as we can."

I heard her, but I didn't *know* what it meant to have a premature baby. I asked, "Can she be born that early?" When I look back, it's a good thing I didn't know that the youngest preemie ever was born only a few days younger at twenty-one weeks and four days. I was a day away from being twenty-two weeks pregnant with Dakota. If I had known that, I probably would have lost my mind, which, with all of the stress, might have made it likely that I would lose my baby. At the same time, knowing that the youngest preemie ever to survive was now a toddler might have given me some solid ground. You know?

Maternal Instincts When Nothing Else Makes Sense

I lay there with my butt propped up, trying to rest. I was asking myself if I'd ever met any people who were born premature. But that train of thought was too much. I started thinking about people I needed to call, like my brothers Darryl and Tokunbo. The three of us grew up trading off who was mothering who. My mind skipped to being eight years old and reaching to catch my little brother running away from me in his diaper, my hands grabbing hold of his chubby arms and him squirming to get loose. I didn't want to trail off into hard thoughts, but when a woman is having a baby and is hurting and scared, she wants her mama. And I had lost mine a long time ago.

2

Binge

When my mom was around, I could see her do all that was necessary to take care of us and herself. Being addicted didn't mean that she wasn't otherwise coherent and in her right frame of mind. I picked up on her good mothering days. If my brother was crying, I knew to ask the questions: Do I need to change his diaper, do I need to feed him, or do I just need to sit next to him and hold him? I couldn't really identify with everything that was going on with my mother's disappearances, but it is very strange and a blessing that as such a young kid, I knew what to do.

East Orange, New Jersey, 1992
Eight-year-old girls don't care nothing about what the rest of the world thinks about their mothers. They just want their

mothers. I remember Mom's thumbs were burned from the friction of the lighter from lighting the pipe. I looked at her cheeks all sunken in from drawing in the smoke. Her body was so frail from the addiction and not eating. She wasn't but five foot two, so petite like me even without the drugs. To see her sick like that just used to do something to me, make me want her more, because it seemed like she was disappearing into the streets and literally disappearing from right in front of me. My twelve-year-old brother, Darryl, saw her absence as his opportunity for freedom, so he took to the streets right behind her, leaving me to take care of my toddler brother, Tokunbo, whenever Mama and Darryl were in the street hustling, smoking, or doing "what they do" for days on end.

I know I have good memories of my childhood tucked away in my head. I remember my mom's signature look in the nineties with her crispy perm, hair flattened into a ponytail, turtleneck tucked in, with jeans over her belly button. She wore those tennis shoes called pumpkin seeds in either white or black. I remember her smile would light up a room. I remember that much now, but for a long time the dark moments overpowered the good.

In our studio apartment on Grove Street, I slept in the closet under the clothes on the floor. I pretended like I was in a tent camping with all of the extras in there. I had a little TV that sat on a little plastic crate where I kept my scratch-and-sniff diary that I called Rosie because it smelled like roses.

One morning I woke to get ready to go to school. Dionne

Maternal Instincts When Nothing Else Makes Sense

Warwick elementary in East Orange was mine, even though I felt kind of lonely and kept to myself most of the time. The daily walk was my routine and even as a little girl, that's something I needed.

I looked around the room that morning and Mama wasn't laid out on the sofa bed with Tokunbo. He was asleep in a soiled diaper with his big toddler belly rising and falling. I was confused, standing there. If she wasn't coming home, why didn't she take me with her like she usually did? What was I supposed to do about my brother? I just stood there inside my closet door, leaning on the frame.

In my head, I heard my mother's oldest sister PopaAuntie's soft-spoken voice that was not as loud and laughing from the gut like the rest of us. "Do what you got to do." I was just a little girl, but popped into action the way any other woman in my family would have. First order of business was to change Tokunbo's soggy diaper. Thank God there were diapers in the apartment. I laid him down on the floor and got that task out of the way.

Then I climbed on top of the counter to get the stale box of cereal out of the cabinet. It was the no-frills white box with big black letters from the government, cheaper than Rice Krispies. I checked to make sure there weren't any roaches. I shook the box around a little and looked inside. If there were roaches, they would come running out, and if they couldn't, they certainly would when I poured the cereal in the bowls.

Now for the milk. Our refrigerator was only five feet tall, not much bigger than me, for our small kitchen. When we had food, it looked like a lot in there, but there wasn't anything in there but some butter that looked pretty orange, and an open can of government peanut butter. No milk.

I was still all about business. I took our bowls one by one to the sink and put some faucet water in there. Tokunbo with his chubby cheeks and tiny little teeth smiled and ate that cereal up like it was SpaghettiOs or something. He didn't know the difference between cereal with milk and cereal with water.

I wasn't supposed to open our door, but I heard a door slam in the hall of our building and thought, *Maybe that's Mama.* I ran to the door and listened, but it was just people leaving for work. I heard the eight o'clock Grove Street bus stop and start again on the street; I knew it was about the time I usually left the house for school. I went ahead and put on my clean sweat suit, the swishy kind everybody wore in the nineties. I put my little raggedy tennis shoes on. I got ready just in case.

"I won go?" Tokunbo knew I was getting ready to go to school and was scared I was going to go and leave him there.

"Shirley not gonna leave you Bo Bo."

Even though I didn't have friends at Dionne Warwick elementary, I liked my teacher, and school is where I got food and attention. I had my own little wooden desk with my books tucked under and in the pocket. It was that feeling little kids have when something is theirs. Looking back, I know that all of the kids felt that way. We were lonely because we didn't talk about our mamas who were all on drugs. We were all going through the same thing, and school was our normal place.

Maternal Instincts When Nothing Else Makes Sense

The one good thing about being out of school was being able to play with Tokunbo; he was a cute, li'l chunky thing with no clothes on and a saggy diaper, running around the apartment. On the radio, the news went off and the music started. I knew the bell had rung and the day was started at school and I got that lonely feeling in the pit of my stomach, like everybody left the party, like everybody started their day and just left me sitting there.

All day Tokunbo and I listened to the radio and that passed the time. I loved it when Naughty by Nature looped back around to being played every hour. That was my song. I was this little thing who swore I was down with them double because Naughty by Nature was from New Jersey. Tokunbo did his li'l toddler stomp to the music, and I did my freestyle dance, just swinging back and forth, hand in the air, "Horray hooooo haaaay hoooooo." Tokunbo had me laughing, stomping around in circles holding one hand close to his body, with his lip sucked in like he was concentrating and just swinging his other arm back and forth like some old man. "Go BooBoo! Go BooBoo!" He was one of those little brown-skin kids you just want to kiss on all the time. Dancing around the apartment with him just took the crazy empty confused feeling away, made it feel like I wasn't waiting.

I was always waiting, though. Just sitting somewhere waiting for Mama. It would be me and other kids, sometimes, sitting in a room, and the grown-ups would be in another room of a two- or three-bedroom apartment. Just gone, high, forgot about their kids. We would play and hang out, jumping and flipping on some old mattresses.

One time it was just me, no other kids, no TV. It wasn't the day of the iPad, just me sitting there, waiting, not knowing how much time went by. Mama was in the bedroom doing her thing getting high, using drugs with other people. Apparently, they didn't have the crack she needed to smoke that day, but she needed to get high right then. So instead of the pipe she shot up with a needle and because that wasn't her drug of choice, she wasn't mentally or physically stable after that. "Come on Shirley. I need to get out of this house." I had learned to just observe, play, and obey.

She was wobbly and disoriented like a drunk as we left. Mind you, I am short now, and was short then too, but my mother wasn't but five feet one inch tall. I wasn't any taller than her, but I had to get her home. Mom was so high it was like walking with somebody who was walking in their sleep.

I don't remember saying anything while we walked. I didn't have a voice. I remember sounds, though. I did a lot of listening while my voice was silent. I remember the sound of the bus, like the air coming out of the hydraulic thing when people were getting on, then the squeaking of the steering wheel, and the brakes when it took off. I remember every time we passed an alley, I smelled piss. I was just there with her out on the street at night and doing what needed to be done.

Maternal Instincts When Nothing Else Makes Sense

I always paid attention to which way we were going, so I knew how to get home. I held her up as we walked over the bridge, and the eight blocks back to our studio apartment. *24 South Grove Street in East Orange, New Jersey, on the first floor, the third door on the left.* I kept repeating it in my head like I practiced in case I ever had to tell an ambulance where we lived. My shoulder hurt and it seemed like those blocks lit by East Orange streetlights with crooked sidewalks went on forever. I didn't care, I was with my mama, helping my mama. I guided her home, holding her up, stopping to keep her from crossing the street, guiding her to step up on the curb, and when we got home, I took her keys out of her purse to open the door.

We got into the apartment that night, and she just lay on the bed. She looked beat down like that part on *Losing Isaiah* when Halle Berry is in the trash can. Her hair was all sticking up and she smelled bad, like piss and old sweat. I was so worried that night. I just took her shoes off and watched her sleep, but at least I was with her.

Tokunbo and I sat down on the sofa bed when the radio commercials came on with men talking too fast about buying cars, and the commercials came one after the other. I just wanted my music back.

The music kept me from having memories so they flooded in without it. I started asking myself, *Why is my mom like this?* My little head was just spinning. I folded up the sofa bed by myself, real slow so it didn't pinch my hand the way it sometimes did. By the time "O.P.P." was playing for the fifth time, I knew I needed to feed me and Tokunbo again, but the cereal was all gone, and I knew I wasn't supposed to leave. Plus, what if she came back?

When it started to get dark, I looked through the little apartment refrigerator and looked in the cabinets. In between I prayed, "God please bring some food." Then I opened the cabinets and refrigerator again. People in the building came home from work, shutting their doors and creaking around on the floor. The smell of onions and fried food was wafting into our apartment, and I got to opening the cabinets and closing them waiting for the magic. Tokunbo played too, laughing and smacking shut the bottom cabinets. The neighbors must have thought my mother was home and we were cooking up a storm, making all of that noise. When the building got quiet with TV sounds and plates clinking, my belly got this sinking feeling in it like I was disappearing like Mama.

The lights on Grove Street flickered in the window, and I had to turn on the lights in the apartment. Thank God the electric bill had been paid. I heard a siren outside and said the prayer I remembered hearing people say at our church, "Father God in Heaven, protect . . ." and I inserted "Mama." I opened my eyes and waited for God to send her walking up Grove.

The hungrier I got, the more confused I felt. I was standing there in the room looking out the window onto the empty sidewalks like I was in some kind of trance.

Maternal Instincts When Nothing Else Makes Sense

I turned off the lights and hid with the TV in my closet bedroom. Tokunbo curled up and went to sleep with me with the Johnny Carson show keeping us company. I wrote in my scratch-and-sniff journal, "Well Rosie, today my mom left again, and I'm mad she did." Tokunbo's breathing went deep, and at least he was sleeping so I could worry about just Mama, but then he woke up. "Shirley, I'm mon eat. I'm mon eat some food."

Then I remembered something. It's funny how instincts aren't part of your reality until something triggers them. Lying on the floor in my closet, I remembered one Christmas, our neighbor Mama Jessie gave me and Tokunbo a real Christmas tree. My brother Darryl brought it in and leaned it against the wall and went back out in the streets. I had some Red Hots and popcorn and decorated the tree, but when Darryl and Mama didn't come back for hours, I picked them off and ate them with Tokunbo.

I didn't break down crying or anything like that, the way any little girl should have. I just did what had to be done, like I was born with some maternal light switch. I got up off the floor, turned the light on, and went into action.

Back in the day we had our people that we clicked with who would always tell us where there were apartments available, people who had our back and we had theirs. Mama Jessie was one of our people. She lived in our building but had lived in the same building as us on two other occasions. Mama always had trouble keeping the lights on and rent paid, so we would move often. Mama would just tell somebody in our welfare network,

"Girl, I have to move out by such and such date. Let me know if you hear of anything that opens up."

I put Tokunbo in a clean diaper and set him on my hip. I knew where to get food. I was like Mama when she used to get us up and get down to the welfare office. She used to say, "Do your business before twelve p.m. Get your food stamps, calculate the groceries, know how much food stamps you have for the month? Budget and don't go over." I was taught the early bird catches the worm, and my mom was very serious about that. She would be up and at the welfare office first thing, and I'd have my shoes on, dressed early, and would be right there with her. That's part of what helps me be the businesswoman I am today, because I was always with her. She used to hold it all up and hold it together until she started getting really far into the addiction and gradually fell apart.

I walked barefoot down to the last door at the end of the hallway to Mama Jessie's. I knocked on the door a few times. I knew that if she didn't answer the door to just knock again because it was late after Johnny Carson went off, so she was probably sleeping in her chair. When I look back, she reminds me of the mother in the movie *Precious* played by Mo'Nique. You know, with a scarf tied to the front with rollers. Mama Jessie might have looked like Precious's mean mama with the housedress, slippers, and that deep scratchy voice, but she was the opposite of mean. She was the sweetest, most nurturing person you'd ever want to meet.

"Hey, baby, what's up. Where your mother at?" The TV flickered on where she had been sitting with a blanket in her chair, and the smell of fried pork chops from hours earlier wafted out into the hall.

I was straightforward. "Hey Mama Jessie. We hungry; I need some food. Can we have some cereal?" If she had it, she'd give what she had to who needed it. If she didn't have it, she'd give you something different. She always looked out for us. She would let Mama run the extension cord if the lights got cut off, and let us use her land line. People would call her phone for us, and she would take a message. I was very comfortable with her.

Today I get a lot of my caretaking, and my mannerisms and way of being, from her. If I have it to share, I'll share it. "Here, beautiful. No problem. You don't owe me anything." If I don't and you are in need, I'll at least call somebody and try to hook you up. Mama Jessie said, "God is always there, and if he can't be there baby, he always have somebody there for you as his replacement."

She gave me an opened box of Cheerios. "Here baby. Take the whole box home." I don't know how she knew we were using faucet water for milk, but she put it in a plastic bag and put a quart of milk in there too. She hung it on my one arm that was holding Tokunbo's butt up on my hip. "Come back down here if you get hungry."

"Yes ma'am."

Mama Jessie was my ram in the bush that night.

I don't know how I knew what to do in that situation. Instincts are amazing. They just kick in if you are in survival mode. But who wants their child pushed to that point? I can't imagine my eight-year-old Demi having to wake up here in this house with her little sisters and me just missing in action, leaving her to call up her maternal survival instincts in order to see herself through to the end of the day.

3

A Baby Story

Premature is considered any baby born younger than thirty-six weeks. If they are born anywhere as young as twenty-five weeks, they have a low survival rate. Dakota was a day shy of twenty-two weeks in my womb.

Dr. Young squeezed my hand. "Well, she's going to be born that early." There was a pause like in playing cards when you have played your hand and are hoping the other players won't put anything lethal on the table.

"Okay." I held on to Dr. Young's hand and asked one more question. "Can you just please continue to be honest with me?"

She smiled. "Can you continue to ask questions rather than yelling at all the nurses?" JR, Dr. Young, and I all chuckled, the first sound of anything that resembled normalcy. As she exited the room, she drew the curtain around JR and me and Dakota in my belly. We stayed like that in our little bubble for only a couple of hours. JR was able to get out his first words to me that didn't have the sounds of nurses cutting in around his thoughts.

"Babe, babe. This is unbelievable, but I'm glad I'm here."

I didn't think I was ever gonna say this, but I told him, "I'm glad you broke your thumb."

He smiled that sleepy smile at me, knowing what I meant. Then, our moment of normal ended when Dr. Young returned. She went over to the little sink, scrubbed her hands, and then put on those blue gloves that I was already sick of looking at. "Before I raise the bed up, I'm going to check your cervix again." She put one blue-gloved hand on the sheet around my knee when she talked to me, the same way she did earlier when holding my hand.

I looked at JR while she poked around down there. I heard her scoot her rolling stool back. She didn't look at me at first, just went to tap her foot on the trash can and toss the gloves in before coming back to hold my hand. She raised her eyes to JR and then down to me. "Honey, it's not looking good. Dakota's feet are right there. She's breech." She just kept talking, like she wanted to get to the assuring part. "But we are going to try. We will try to keep her up there for as long as possible. She might turn around on her own."

She pulled the curtain back around us, and JR and I were just quiet, trying to hold on to each other while trying to deal with what we were hearing. A nurse came in and attached a drug to my IV bag to stop the contractions. Then another drip for a light dose of pain medicine. I watched her like I used to watch the pigeons outside of the apartment window when I was a kid, trying to ground myself in their busy movements until my mother came home.

I looked at JR and he was just holding my hand, like he was waiting for me to say something. "Babe. It's gonna be okay," he said, and I started crying. I didn't even know at that point if I was registering it all, but the tears were a release; couldn't nothing else happen with all of that but tears.

He looked helpless, too. "I'm gonna get you some ice chips." He needed to do something, anything to make it better.

He put the ice chips in my mouth and it felt good to have his hand to my lips; the ice tasted like salt with my tears. He adjusted the pillow under my butt to help keep me elevated. Every now and then he just said, "Babe, it's gonna be okay," and somewhere in there, I fell asleep.

I woke up just past dusk to the smell of hospital dinners and the sight of the dark room and all those little glowing green lights on everything. The inside of my mouth was burning like I was holding a mouthful of hot coffee.

I turned to see JR's silhouette sleeping in the chair. I said, "Babe, I'm hot." He leaned forward, put his hand on my forehead, and immediately picked up the nurses' button near my bed.

Through the night, they gave me light meds to bring down the fever. By noon the next day, the nurses said they were going to have to break my water. I was twenty-two weeks exactly that day. It was still too early. I got an attitude. "No! That's going to make her come out! I thought the point was to keep her in there, that all I had to do was keep my butt elevated and count the days. I can do that."

I didn't understand that they needed to break my water to test it for infection. I didn't understand that having a fever that wouldn't go down put them in emergency mode. I kept protesting, but three of them in their aqua scrubs rolled a tray of gadgets in, put those blue gloves on, and the next thing I knew, I felt pressure where they stuck something in my vagina like I was getting my yearly exam.

It was quiet for a second, and one of them asked in a low voice, "Is the fluid green?" and another one said, "She has an infection." They were lifting my bottom to change the pad under me, and I saw a little of the green stuff. Things were wavering again, like the night two nights before when I was on the couch; I was struggling to keep my eyes open. One of them took a swab of some of the green stuff and put it in a long tube. I saw the IV bag being messed with again. I heard them tell JR "group beta strep." I felt them rolling me over and I held JR's muscular arm while they gave me a shot in the butt, and I fell asleep for what must have been another hour.

Group beta strep is an infection that pregnant women have that is normally dormant—like so many other diseases that Black women end up with. It's dormant, but a stressful life is like the alarm clock that wakes it up. That afternoon, Dr. Young explained to me and JR that they usually test for it in every pregnant woman around her thirty-fifth week, but I didn't make it anywhere near that.

JR asked the questions, his eyes barely open, like exhaustion was about to take him down. "Is it dangerous?"

Dr. Young kept her promise to be honest. "It can be deadly, but Shirley is already here in the hospital. She's already on meds."

"What about Dakota? Does she have it?"

"She's running the risk of having the infection, too."

That's when the thoughts got to rolling. *Why?* When I was pregnant with Demi, I was fine. *How did I get this?* When I first moved to Ohio there was a period of time when I was unin-sured, and I had an abnormal Pap smear. I had to have a colpos-copy through some jankedy insurance at my clinic. Maybe all the scraping they did in my uterus left me vulnerable? I had no idea but my thoughts were running absolutely wild, wondering if I had somehow caused this even accidentally.

Dr. Young responded like she could hear me thinking. "There's no explanation why it shows up in some pregnant women and not in others." At the time, that's all doctors knew. It was a mystery why women of color, or women who had it hard from the get-go, got things like group beta strep and preeclampsia while pregnant. Doesn't even matter if you had it hard and life got better, some illnesses just be in there waiting for stress to set them off. It doesn't matter that childbirth can be celebra-tory good stress. The body doesn't understand good stress. It just feels the stress, thinks the hard times are coming again and breaks down, no matter how much money you have in the bank.

She paused and took a breath before saying, "Shirley, JR. We are going to take Dakota."

I pleaded, "Please don't take her. I want to have a natural childbirth."

JR cut in. "Dakota may not have the infection, and then we're taking her when she should have stayed in."

Dr. Young remained calm, but her voice became stern. "The risk is high. We'd have to monitor you and her every ten minutes and she's in distress already, and we sure can't do anything to save her if she passes in utero."

While we were arguing with Dr. Young, my ears latched on to one nurse's question to JR. "Have you thought about funeral arrangements for Dakota, or do you want something quiet with the family here?" For a moment, I asked myself if I was delusional. I hadn't slept and felt like I was barely holding on to my sanity. *Did I hear this woman ask my husband about funeral arrangements for my baby?* I blurted out, "Don't nobody else come in here talking death about my daughter! Everybody, get out of here! I don't want nobody but Dr. Young talkin to me!"

Dr. Young shooed everyone out of the room and gave us a few minutes to process everything. I had JR put on gospel music to keep me calm, "I Need You to Survive" by Hezekiah Walker: "You are important to me, I need you to survive. I need you, you need me."

Maternal Instincts When Nothing Else Makes Sense

I held my hands on my quiet belly and was praying to Dakota's spirit, and to God, for the two of them to be of one accord. I knew if she could stay, that I could feed her, take care of her, I could weather any storm for her. I just needed her to survive. Life broke my mother, but I had survived to be a good mother for my daughters. *If you can survive, Dakota, I can do the rest, just survive. I need you to survive. I love you. Dakota, I need you to be here.* JR and I prayed her up, inside my womb. Holding the space open between life and death until we were spent and could let God take hold.

Dr. Young came back in the room and whispered, "Okay, we will leave her in, and check you every ten or fifteen minutes. Shirley, don't hesitate to push that button if something doesn't feel right."

In my memory, it seemed like days later, but it was only a couple of hours later, around five o'clock on my second day in the hospital. It was the day that JR had an appointment to get his cast taken off. His doctor was going to be at the arena only that day, and it took less than an hour to get a cast cut off. He kept saying, "That can wait," but I told him, "Nothing is happening but me lying here with my butt up in the air. Do something normal, even if it's getting the cast off. Just go and come back."

As soon as he left, I felt so hot it was like my brain was melting. I pressed the nurse's button.

Dr. Young came right back in the room. My fever was spiking

again. She said, "Shirley, it's you or your baby. I know you want to wait, but the wait is over. You are sick. You need to agree to let me take her."

All the things that happened seemed impossible in such a short period of time. I called JR. "Honey, you have to come back. They are going to induce labor." Nurses came and lowered the bed, put Pitocin in my IV. Dr. Young checked my cervix.

I had sent JR away, trying to be all brave and keep things normal. He had missed Demi's birth eight years ago because he had a game that day. I needed him. I needed somebody. I put my thoughts on Dakota. *God, please let Dakota live.* I wasn't thinking about my own life, just hers. They took my hands off my belly and guided me to wrap them around the plastic bed rails to keep them out of Dr. Young's way.

That's when I felt something wet on my left side. I told Dr. Young, "Can you look and make sure I didn't pee on myself?" She was in get-shit-done mode. She didn't smile or put her hand on my hand but pulled up her little rolling stool, put one glove on, and said, "She's hemorrhaging." I remember my cousin Lynette saying she was hemorrhaging every time she was on her period. I could tell this was different.

Ambulance sirens were going off in my head: *hemorrhaging.* Dr. Young yelled it this time, "She's hemorrhaging!" She was looking at me but talking to the nurses and to anybody in earshot who could get in the room and help. She tried to hold my gaze, looking up at me from between my parted legs over her glasses. I knew in that moment that she was looking to make sure my eyes were still open.

Everything was surreal: People came in with one type of cart and another. I lost what seemed like short snippets of time, like I would blink and somebody who was standing next to me would then be down next to Dr. Young. I smelled a familiar soap like lavender and looked over and there was my best friend from high school, Kawana. I had known that tall brown girl since tenth grade and we never had a single fight. She was like an angel in my life, such a pure, easygoing spirit; she knew my struggle. I don't remember her getting there, so I thought God had sent her. She had her hand over my left hand. That's when I realized Ma was on my right side with her hand over my other hand.

Dr. Young's voice got supercalm, which let me know death was in the room. "Shirley, we want you to push soon."

I was protective and delirious at the same time. "No! She has to stay in there."

Then Dr. Young was done with her calm voice. She spoke quickly and sternly: "Shirley, we need to go ahead and take Dakota. You have Demi and your husband, so we can't lose you." I finally understood. Dr. Young's demeanor was like my mother's sisters'; they could listen and play nice, but when shit needed to happen, they would snatch me into place.

The next thing I knew, I was lying there, looking to the

side at Kawana again. I held my eyes on her eyes. I could hear Dr. Young's direct tone, giving instructions. The nurses were whisper-chatting, trying to prepare me for the worst. "Shirley, Dakota won't make it. Her eyes won't be open when you look at her. Okay?" I felt the push coming. At that very moment, JR, Pop, and Dimitrius burst into the room and moved the curtain. I could see them in my peripheral vision, but I was locked there staring at Kawana. I could feel JR and his family and Dr. Young, and I knew Dakota and I were being intentionally held in this life.

I felt my whole body curl into two quick pushes, and Dakota came out. I whispered to Kawana, "I'm too scared to look."

Then God said, *Look at her.* I couldn't look. God said, *Look at her.* I turned my head and saw these black beady ant eyes and in them a reflection of my eyes and my mother's eyes the day she died, and I broke down crying uncontrollably and looked away.

I felt JR kissing my forehead and everybody in the room whispered, "Look at her, Shirley. Look at her before they take her away." The grief was so intense that I couldn't turn my head. I couldn't even make a sound, but I followed Kawana's eyes to where they held Dakota in their gaze.

My brain detached to save itself from what didn't make sense, the sight of Dakota's body outside of my body, here, and yet not here. I saw the nurses scoop this tiny being in something like Saran Wrap. She didn't even have skin yet. JR cut the cord without touching her or disturbing the plastic. Dakota Ida Smith, one pound, stared out into the room at 6:56 p.m. looking for her mother. But her naked silhouette was wrapped up and gone from my sight and my touch. She was alive, that was the most important thing, she was alive.

Dropping Jewels

Repairing Maternal Instincts Interrupted by Disease, Drugs, and Poverty

In the moments after Dakota was born and seeing her for the first time, I felt a disconnect, like my knowledge bank was empty, because this was different. It was a situation I was *not* familiar with. Before having a premature baby, I felt like I was the mother of everyone, even my mother. I had an older daughter, had raised my brother; I knew how this went. But I didn't know anything about premature birth even though I knew so much about mothering from an early age. I had to tell myself, *Shirley, you got this. You always been somebody's mother. You have to draw on that experience the best you can. When the time comes to know what to do next, you will know.*

I did know what to do about some things, like to tell everybody to shut up and let me focus on prayer. But so many things I didn't know. My instincts had been interrupted early in life by a need to kick into maternal survival mode when I was just a baby myself.

I was a Black girl with a mom addicted to drugs, alcohol, crack cocaine, pills. There are all sorts of drugs out there that are attractive to Black mothers with children, fathers missing, a household to keep up, women who are basically set up by society to fail.

According to the *New York Times*, by December 16, 1990, the majority of the ten thousand reported AIDS cases in the state of New Jersey were in Newark; of those cases 53 percent were diagnosed as intravenous drug users. In the nineties, my mother was a victim of both diseases, addiction and HIV/AIDS.

But little Black girls don't know anything about all of that. As a little girl you just look up to your mom, especially if you don't have your dad on the scene. I looked up to my mom so much. I didn't even know who my real dad was until later in life. Our moms are our heroes. She is the first person you see when you come out.

If she goes missing, it is like your bread going missing. How can you survive that? How can you draw on maternal instincts that have been so interrupted in their formation?

When those drugs come between a mother and daughter, it takes away a Black girl's mother-hero and it takes a whole lifetime to repair that damage. That is, if you get time to repair it. When the foundation is broken between mother and daughter, it's a hard puzzle to put back together.

Here's some advice I offer the women out there to help them regain their instincts:

Maternal Instincts When Nothing Else Makes Sense

- Know that you have instincts coming out of your behind. You have survived so much that resilience is your knowledge.

- You have to stop doubting yourself. It's less that your instincts have been interrupted than that your belief in your instincts has been interrupted.

Here is some information I tell mothers to help them put the pieces of the puzzle back together when their maternal development was interrupted by their own mom being absent because of addiction to drugs and substances:

- Please understand that she does not want to be that way.

- Please love your mother unconditionally as best as you can in each stage that she is in.

- Remember, it's the disease that's taking her away from being the person she was called to be.

- Those times when she came out of it and tried to compensate, that's because she knew that when she was in it, she was not her best self.

- Love her, she needs it.

PART II

Community as the Fish
and the Loaves of Bread

No matter how long I was told to be strong as a Black woman, I knew that even when I was a little girl, part of being strong was being brave enough to ask for help from my community. When I was growing up, there was a community of other folks on public assistance who shared information on where to move next for Section 8 housing, where to get the most food for your food stamp dollar, and so on. I was a kid and didn't even know the power of that word-of-mouth underground community that helped my mother navigate a system of rules designed to keep her and her children in poverty. At thirty-six I'm just peeling back the layers of understanding that Black mothers have to grow up with a lot. Just being Black alone comes with the implanted idea that you have to be a strong hustler to navigate around systemic racism.

I'm just now really seeing what all this has meant in my life and seeing all the other hustlers in my community who kept me afloat. Community showed up for me when I gave birth to Dakota and the shit was hitting the fan.

4

Liquid Gold

Mama Jessie taught me that as long as you have community, there is no need for anybody to ever go hungry.

I didn't carry Dakota to term. They had to take her from my body to save us both, and I still had a severe infection to deal with. How was I supposed to produce milk? On the day she was born, I just sat all night in the dark. Nurses came in and out. Fluorescent light flowed in from the hallway. All those beeping sounds and blue lights and numbers glowed in the dark of my room. We had been sitting down to New Year's Eve dinner, and in three days, things had gone from sugar to shit.

All I knew was to talk to God. "God, you wouldn't bring me this situation if it wasn't for a reason."

Mama Bear

Over the next couple of days my infection started to go away, my mind started to register what had happened. People gave me literature to read, and I tried to take in the words in the brochures about preemies and life expectancy, but nothing was going through my mind at that point but guilt. *What did I do wrong? I should have had a healthier diet, shouldn't have gone places, been so active.* I was stuck.

The hospital had a room across from the NICU that JR and I could rent out for a maximum of a week, and we did. There was a bed and a bathroom. Me and JR held that space every day that was allowed. The nurses started asking me if I could produce milk. I was feeling the pressure of what everybody kept saying, that breast milk is the best for Dakota. I tried to eat well, drink lots of water, tried to sleep and get rest in hope that my milk would come.

Everybody and their granma had advice and I just wanted everybody to shut up. Of course, I couldn't produce milk. My tiddies didn't even blow up. I had carried only a couple of days past being four months pregnant. What the hell were they thinking by giving me breast milk advice? It was like they were ignoring the reality of the situation and making the guilt worse by acting like the reason I wasn't giving milk was because I wasn't drinking enough water or eating right. I never felt so useless in my life. My baby was down the hall struggling and I couldn't do anything to feed her. I was just running around in my head trying to think of solutions. I had nothing. Even when I drank a bunch of water, I would only get a teardrop of milk. They would put it on a Q-tip and rub it on Dakota's fragile little lips, which were no bigger than the tip of my pinky fingernail.

They told me Dakota was still losing ounces. She was disappearing before I ever got to hold her. There was more talk of death and her funeral. She lay there, smaller than my own hand, flesh of my flesh struggling for her life, and me and JR couldn't do anything but watch. It was like all of us were dying.

Everybody in the basketball community was being supportive and trying to let each other know what was happening so they could be a strong network for us. On our last morning in the rented hospital room, Afra—I call her Affy—came to visit. She is the wife of one of JR's teammates. She is a woman who has a glow to her. She is one of those people who lights up the room with her smile the way my mother used to. But she is also smart and informed, hands-on with her children, and a great wife.

She had been nine months pregnant when I was four months and had just given birth to her son. She brought me a fruit basket with healthy grains and drinks. I told her I wasn't able to produce milk. She saw how stressed out that made me and reminded me that this was her second child. She said in her British accent, "Darling each time my milk comes it's like liquid gold. You see how I eat organic. We are family. I have milk for your baby and mine."

She listened to the whole status of Dakota's weight dropping and didn't roll into giving me advice about how to make my body do the impossible. Like it wasn't even in question, she said, "Oh yes, Mommy. We are going to turn that around." I talked to JR about it, he said, "Word! Yes."

I talked to one of the nurses about it and she said, "The hospital gets donated milk. It has to be screened; you can't just get it straight from another woman." By the time the hospital washed donor milk, it was free of the nutrients that could help Dakota put on weight and survive. It would be like feeding her water while watching her die.

After a week of renting the family room, JR and I knew it was time to go. The anxiety hit. Leave, what the hell is that? I knew I had another child. I had to jump back in with Demi. But I couldn't wrap my mind around leaving. I was so anxious; my heart was racing. They had cameras in the NICU where I could log in and see Dakota, but leave her? No! It was so hard, not like going to get fresh air for just a minute. Intentionally leaving her made me feel like I was giving up.

The first time I left the hospital, I took Demi to school and came right back. The separation was too much to bear even though I had never held my Dakota. When I was driving back from Demi's school, I kept thinking, *Is she okay, are they treating her okay, will she not feel my presence and realize I'm not in the room? In the two hours I'm gone will she take a turn for the worse? Damn! How do I do this?*

Dakota was only a couple of weeks old. The hospital staff was urging us to move into a new normal. I didn't want to be selfish to other families who needed the family room. Our turn was over, and we needed to deal with our new lives. If it wasn't for them gently telling me I didn't have a choice but to go home to my own bed, I don't think I would have ever left. I was a mess.

The anxiety of being removed from Dakota every night made it clear to me that I needed to do whatever was necessary to get Dakota strong enough to come home. I wasn't even thinking about rules and following them or breaking them. I stopped considering the rules and followed my instincts. I did what I needed to do for my child's survival.

Affy, her husband, her three-year-old, and her brand-new baby lived near Demi's school. So in the morning I dropped Demi off at school and drove over to their house. I made coffee and played with her toddler and bounced her newborn while she pumped liquid gold. She was selfless, and I needed that.

Dressed in my daily wear of sweatpants, sneakers with no socks, T-shirt, and a ball cap, I took the pumped milk and my writing notebooks for my day at the hospital. I told myself, *Fret not*, and walked right into the NICU to feed my Dakota.

I smiled at those nurses with "my" milk labeled like I had pumped it. I heard God say that the rules about donor milk were the rules of man, not his rules. So I told the lie loud enough for the nurses to hear me, "Good morning, Dakota Bear. Time for Mommy's milk."

Affy and I did this for three weeks, and I thank God for her and her love; I knew to ask and listen to my instincts, to stop doubting. I knew that Affy was the community I needed to step in, to listen and do. Dakota gained her first solid pound on that liquid gold.

5

Reaching Out to My Othermothers

Community can be defined in all kinds of ways, from the sistah who sees you can't feed your child because your milk hasn't come in, to the neighbor who is the only one in the building who has paid her phone bill and becomes the lifeline for all the neighbors who need to dial out for help. Then there is the community that sits right in front of us. If you sift through your family members, there are always the ones standing right there, who have been there all of your life, ready to pitch in.

That week Mama was on a binge and didn't come home, I lost count of how many nights she was gone, maybe a week. Every morning the sofa was still folded up and the bathroom door was unlocked and open. I lost track of the number of times it got dark, the number of times I prayed, and the number of times

I asked Mama Jessie for food for me and Tokunbo, but I do remember that I had missed a lot of school and that made me mad. Being pissed off must have been some kind of motivation, because one morning I put Tokunbo back on my hip, walked to Mama Jessie's, and called PopaAuntie, my mother's oldest sister, Kim.

Her number was scribbled on the wall next to our phone mount. The phone didn't work and was one of Tokunbo's toys. I have always been good with remembering numbers. I chanted the number all the way down to Mama Jessie's with Tokunbo saying back all kinds of numbers that almost confused me, "973–373 . . ." I rehearsed what I would say. "PopaAuntie can you come get me and Tokunbo? I don't know where Mama and Darryl are."

I had to keep it stepping down the hall with Tokunbo on my hip while keeping PopaAuntie's number in my head. I was also trying to rehearse what to say and how much to say. I was already stuck in the woman-dilemma of when to speak and when to stay quiet. I didn't want PopaAuntie to think anything bad about her favorite sister. I imagined her saying "Lord!" in her soft-toned way and shaking her head the way she did in church, but I was also thinking maybe she wouldn't believe me, or think I was exaggerating.

I told PopaAuntie just the bare minimum. "Can you come and get us? Mama and Darryl aren't home." She sent her daughter Lynette, my oldest cousin, who was seventeen years old at the time but grown by the standard of the women in our family.

I didn't know to tell Lynette that Mama had been gone for days. So she didn't know any better than to hang on to me for the weekend and bring me back to the apartment Sunday night, where I was glad to find Mama sleeping like the whole thing never happened. After that binge, even the abnormal in my life didn't have a rhythm to it.

Word on the streets travels faster than the Word in the church. Well slightly faster, because both will make your head spin. I guess word got around on the street that Mama was using, because Tokunbo's father, who Mama had done wrong over her addiction, came and picked up his son.

It was just me and Mama then, and we did a lot of walking to chase her high, because we didn't even have money for the bus and I wasn't going anywhere without her, so I walked. It didn't matter how far away home was, sometimes we were right in the neighborhood, other times we might be as far away as Newark and would have to walk the three miles through the night-time streets, under the highway, just walking like we were in an urban migration or something. My LA Gears were already raggedy, and we did so much walking, I about wore them down to nothing.

It was a long time, maybe four years, that I was either following Mama to whatever drug house or I was just left behind at home. Those four years are a blur. I call them the gap.

At some point I went with Mama to live at her twin sister Aunt Anita's house. I don't remember us moving there. Mama was still using. I do remember that they were always having family gatherings and all of my cousins would be in the basement. I know that some days I went to school, some days I didn't. Sometimes Erics, the man who I thought was my father, spent time with me, sometimes he didn't. I know I used to ask him to take me to a few spots on Grove Street to look for Mama because sometimes Mama wouldn't be at Aunt Anita's, so I figured she must be somewhere back in the old neighborhood. We would wait around and nothing.

One day when I was around eleven years old, I was with Erics in Irvington Center, and doing my thing, or rather I was being the object that some adult was just dragging around. I stood in the store, no voice, just present, staring at the bulletproof glass, looking behind the counter at all of the patterns of red and green and white that the cigarette packages made stacked on the shelf. I heard a familiar voice. "Shirley?"

Lynette told me she didn't see me; she recognized my father and figured the dirty child with her hair all messed up and pale blotches on her face must have been me. "Shirley? Is that you?" I barely recognized her. She said she was just stopping in a store to get a Snapple on a hot-ass day, and there I was looking so rundown and bad. My hair was in nappy ponytails, but it didn't matter because the hair band wasn't holding it together; the matted tangle of my hair held things in place.

She started coming to pick me up once a week, which was the most consistency I had for a long time. She fixed me up the best she could each weekend and took me to our family church, Bethlehem Baptist Church in North Newark. As far as the rest of the family knew, she was just bringing her little cousin to church on Sunday, nobody knew all of what my eyes were seeing every day.

One time when she came to get me, she said, "Something ain't right Shirley. I can't take you back over there." Meaning she couldn't take me back to the dark feeling that lingered in my Aunt Anita's house. She didn't know what was happening over there, and I was just used to being drug around, so I didn't know to open my mouth and say something.

The adults knew all of the craziness that was happening in their lives with hustling for money, hustling for drugs, hustling to get up next to God every Sunday. All I had was my perspective, which was, *Go with Daddy. Go with Lynette. Go with Mama.* That's what any child has to go through, no say over where they going or who with. But I was also tired all the time and scared most of the time. It was like Lynette's intuition said to take me home with her. I didn't have a voice but was glad that the right person was making me follow them the right way.

She was twenty-one by then, had a daughter, my four-year-old cousin Kimberly, and still lived with her mother, my Popa-Auntie. She was everybody's rock in our family. PopaAuntie's house was where anybody came if things were hard.

On the day I was born, August 8, 1984, my mom was living with PopaAuntie and began having severe contractions. My aunts tell the story that Mama was having so much pain in her stomach and back, and was like, "Kim take me to the hospital!" My aunt Kim drove over superbumpy potholes of the streets of Newark doing the best she could to keep my head from banging against my mother's bony pelvis. Mama was complaining, "Can you stop driving crazy?"

When they got to the hospital, the nurses gave PopaAuntie scrubs. She was in a panic like a nervous father. "I'm not going in there." PopaAuntie is not a fan of hospitals, but she was not leaving my mother's side. I was carried to full term and birthed at Beth Israel Hospital in Newark, weighing in at six pounds and five ounces.

When PopaAuntie was telling my great-aunt Frances the story back then about being forced to stay in the delivery room, Aunt Frances replied, "Go head popa auntie" and the nickname stuck. I call her PopaAuntie and she calls me Pop. She still has the outfit and the scrub cap today; I don't know what she did with her shoes, though. PopaAuntie told me when I came out I was having a bowel movement. They had to make sure the stool didn't come up in my lungs and it didn't; I crapped on PopaAuntie's right shoe, marking her ass mine.

The first night was very routine. Lynette was like, "Shirley, lay out your clothes on the radiator. Go on in there with Kimberly and y'all both get a bath." I fell right in line, because that's how it was at PopaAutie's house. There were my cousins Billy and

Michael who slept in one room, PopaAuntie had her room, and me and Lynette and my cousin Kimberly shared the queen-size bed in Lynette's room. You know that feeling when you scooch in the middle of people you love, and you are just cozy all in it? It was like that. Everything that I didn't know was supposed to be the life of a twelve-year-old was suddenly in my life.

In the morning, me and Kimberly got to the kitchen and sat down to eat our cereal. Lynette clapped her hands. "Rock and roll, rock and roll y'all, five minutes. Let's go." She walked around the kitchen with her peppy attitude. I wasn't used to that type of organization, but it made me feel like I was a part of their family. She was rushing around the kitchen in her lab coat with her round butt shaping it out in the back the way a Black woman can. She was in a good mood, and smelled good too, like detergent and baby powder and soap. Finally, the smell of the crack pipe was gone.

I washed our dishes and we were out of the house. Lynette took Kimberly to the YMCA for preschool. Then Lynette was off to work coding at a doctor's office. She always had jobs like that and has always been organized. I walked the five and a half blocks to school in Irvington to Myrtle Avenue's Middle School. I felt clean and organized, same old clothes but they were clean. The streets over in Irvington were clean too. I didn't have to walk past the smell of piss and crack fiends.

One girl came out on her stoop. "Hey, walk with us." Just like that. I was with a bunch of seventh graders walking to school. It was just friendly and pure. "What y'all watch on TV last night?" Not that unsafe feeling of watching your back that was starting to happen on the way to my school in East Orange.

For the rest of that week, I was just excited. One of my new homies walked up to the door one morning and was like, "Hey Shirley you ready?" The next morning, I stopped at my new friend Erica's house. "Girl you ready?" The group of kids met up every morning as we walked. It was like I was waking up, like my mind was working again, like whatever stupor I was in was lifted and I was a kid again.

I didn't realize that I was still looking a little raggedy for a middle schooler, and didn't really care. I was just happy, until one day, Lynette was like, "Girl, you still be wearing wrinkled-ass clothes like back in the day. I have to teach you how to iron." The two of us cracked up, and I could hear my mother's voice too. She was always part of making the family joke of *Shirley don't like to iron*. We would go to the laundromat and when we came home, I would not be trying to iron. I would just take the clothes that looked like a balled-up potato-chip bag and put them on. My mother, on the other hand, loved to iron. Her pants would have such tight creases in them that you could put them in the dryer and they would still hold the crease from the previous ironing.

My laugh died down, remembering Mama. Lynette said, "You know I'm just messing with you the way we do. Let's go buy you some new clothes," and that set me right back in a good mood. At the end of my first month with her, she took her check and took me shopping for clothes at Shoppers World in

Elizabeth. I got Reeboks and Reebok Classics. This was back when Toys R Us had Kids R Us. You could walk into one store and get a middle schooler's whole outfit in one place. I never had the experience of shopping for school clothes and my eyes were wide open. It was like eating at a buffet when you ain't seen nothing but an empty refrigerator for weeks.

At night I prayed for God to look over Mama and prayed for her to forgive me for leaving her out there. Kids are kids, though. I was swept up by a member of my family, another mother. I was along for the ride in the batch of family kids. When I look back on it, I'm sure I missed my mother terribly. I even remember still looking for her in the streets and asking to go back to find her, but my growing up moved forward and I lost track of her.

Every morning, I was excited to wake up for school, because I loved school and looked as fresh in my outfit as my little crew. My favorite teacher was Mrs. Zadlock, a white lady who wore that same outdated eighties hairdo as PopaAuntie, short in the front but long in the back. She was my homeroom teacher. She was so nice, had a soft voice that was always understanding. I took to her immediately, which really helped me settle in. I was a taskmaster getting my homework done to get that positive praise. Then I joined the school choir and cheerleading. I had such a positive attitude and just wanted to be friends with everybody.

Me and my girls would always be like, "I'll see you at lunch," "You want me to go over your house or you over mine?" God was putting friendships in my life at the time that just seemed like the fun-loving good time of being young, but it was the start of friendships with girls who grew into the women in my life. It was a time in my life that solidified my ability to make community and friends, especially when shit is hitting the fan.

6

Creating Community Through Social Media

I'm always talking about things going from sugar to shit, but having my cousin Lynette pull me up out of a bad place and becoming a teenager who could make the best of any situation is when I learned to flip things from shit to sugar. I learned to find family and community wherever I was, especially if I was in a bad place or if I couldn't get to my usual people. That's what I leaned on in those days in the NICU, where every day is a roller coaster and you think you are alone without community. I put my skills in place and, with my cousin Danica's help, I used my writing to reach beyond the walls of the hospital.

Mama Bear

For the first few months after Dakota's birth, the NICU became a second home for me, JR, and Demi. I got to know Dakota's nurses personally as they all rooted for the youngest infant to ever take on that preemie battle in Cleveland Clinic's NICU. I also formed some deep bonds with other families who came and went from the NICU. We would share in each other's journeys and offer each other support that only families of preterm babies can offer. It was so strange to be there for so long that I became a kind of constant, like it was a daily job and families would get to know me and go home with their babies after a while and, sadly, some of them would not. I would have community for some days, but then I was alone in this thing again. How can I stay grounded? How can I connect with these other families out there?

I took community to a whole new level with those questions. I had been writing in my journal a lot and my cousin Danica said to me one day, "Shirley, you should start a blog. The jewels of wisdom you drop on these NICU families walks out the door when they take their babies home. A lot of folks could be getting your words." She was right, and I also needed something to ground myself in this experience, something to push the experience out beyond myself. I knew God didn't give me and my family this struggle for no reason, and the idea of blogging would give me purpose.

Danica had the technical know-how. She set up my blog My Kota Bear (https://www.mykotabear.com/blog) and there I was, every day, writing in my journal as a blog not only for the families to benefit, but as a place to put each of the moments that needed to be witnessed.

My very first entry:

I did not see this day coming and when it did it hit like a ton of bricks. So many questions and emotions going on in my head at one time, I went from one extreme to another in the blink of an eye. One tear quickly turned into millions and at that point all I could do is pray. Who am I to question God? Nobody! So I didn't. However, that did not mean that I wasn't angry, hurt, confused, and disappointed with myself and the curveball that life just threw me.

Everything happened so fast that it is still taking some time to fully understand and swallow this huge pill. I am still processing the birth of Dakota and I'm sure I will do so for a while because there are so many questions that I have. I kept telling myself "It's my fault"; I felt the urgent need to blame someone so I chose ME!

My brain is going and going just like the Energizer bunny, so much that I cannot rest or sleep. We went from celebrating the holidays with family and friends to a sudden life change overnight. Our lives have been switched to a minute-by-minute situation and we must learn how to adjust our clocks for the days, weeks, and months ahead.

For all of the families who have been through this journey before us we thank you in advance for leading us and helping us get through this critical time. For the families who are going through this journey right now we are one with you. We stand, touch, and agree that your child will be healed beyond human comprehension. Last but not least, for the families that will have the misfortune of living in and going through this journey, I can only hope and pray that a small piece of our story can help you in the time of need as you learn how to live minute by minute.

We would like to wish our God-sent daughter Dakota Smith a happy birthday. May God keep you and bless you in all the days of your life.

From my heart to yours.

The preemie and NICU experience is a world inside of and outside of the larger world. Folks need community in that experience that is like none other. My social media started blowing up with families who just needed that connection, needed to know they weren't alone as I shared the good days and the hellish days. And it gave us a boost to keep going as a family when we received tweets from Cavalier fans who spoke of ways Dakota's journey and our faith in God gave them the strength to carry on in the face of all kinds of life-or-death circumstances.

It was the beginning of February and I started feeling like there was light at the end of the tunnel. I woke up a little more chipper. Afra's breast milk was one of the big shifts. I could see the miracle happen where they had said in the NICU there would be mostly bad days. My cousin's help with the blog was a big shift, and JR and I standing together in our decision to post pictures of our experience was a big shift. It put us out there. Folks were seeing our pains and joys inside the nooks and crannies, but it was making a difference. We had taken the gifts given to us by Afra and Danica and were giving back that life to other families just by sharing our truth. I had spent a lot of days sitting in the NICU wondering what God's purpose for me in this situation was. What was the purpose of me having these hardships in my life? To be honest, I had always struggled with my purpose, but blogging was leading me back to the way I had always dealt with struggles: writing. I prayed that my blog and social media writings would somehow create a support system for others. It was doing just that and more. I had a following that I felt so connected to, it was unreal, and when I blogged, my readers requested more; they were always hungry to read more. That is when I thought to myself, *Maybe my purpose is to be an author.*

As I worked to balance being in the NICU and being there for Demi and being a good wife, I took little moments to myself here and there, stealing time whenever I was running an errand for Demi. It was time to just think for a moment outside of the NICU without guilt. On Fridays, Demi had a gymnastics class from 4:15 to 6:30, and I would go to a nearby sushi bar there in Broadview Heights around the corner from our house. I told myself not to feel guilty. It was either sit for an hour waiting for Demi to finish, which meant I wasn't in the NICU with Dakota but was worrying myself to death, or spend the time catching my breath.

Mama Bear

One day, I packed a book in my bag, *Present over Perfect: Leaving Behind Frantic for a Simpler, More Soulful Way of Living.* It was a book my photographer friend Brittany, who took Dakota's preemie pictures, had given me while I was in the NICU. I stopped at the sushi bar, ordered, and while sitting there at the counter waiting, I started reading Shauna Niequist's story. She had made her life too busy and was trying to be too perfect; but she did not allow herself to be still enough to enjoy this existence. I was relating to her story in the first few pages.

I inserted my bookmark to be sure not to lose my page. I laid my book on the bar and picked up my cell phone and began to text JR: "Babe, I think I want to write, like really be an author because the more books I read it keeps nudging at me. When I read these different books I think to myself shit I can write too. lol what do you think?" I placed my phone back down and thought to myself, *Shirley, what in the world did you just text your husband? He's gonna think you losing it.* I picked the book back up, and a few minutes later I heard JR's text alert sound off. I was so anxious to read his reply I snatched my phone off the bar and read, "I agree!" I stared in a daze for a few seconds like something was waking up in me. I could feel what it felt like to have a sense of purpose. I picked up my book and kept reading.

God had put us through this for a reason, there was some purpose. Who were we to hold this moment in secret when there were other families going through the same thing and needing some light? My and JR's social media family got to witness our struggle and hold vigil for us while holding out hope for their own children. I admit, it wasn't just an act to help other folks like some martyr, I was also in need. That's what community can be like, you need something and when you are providing for others you are fulfilling that need.

The blogging and social media posts started out as a way to keep talking to folks as if they were there in the NICU for 141 days with me and my family. It was a way to be grounded and not feel isolated. I didn't know at the time that it was a way to connect across the country with families who were needing community and relief from the isolation as much as I was needing it. Making community just requires us to reach out, whether it's to ask for help or to offer it or to vent and write our stories. From childhood to now, I have learned that the courage to write down my truth and to reach out helps me to see that I'm not alone, and I always find that God has put somebody right there to reach for my hand.

Dropping Jewels

Advice for Families Who
Are Feeling Alone

It has been a big part of Black women's history to construct community out of who and what we have available. Back in the day and even now, our families, our schools, churches, beauty shops, and more have Black women at the helm, holding everybody together as community. PopaAuntie and Mama Jessie played that role in my early life; Bishop Glanton holds that community leader position in my church; and I chose to create and hold space as that person in my NICU community in New Jersey by creating a nonprofit to help support families with preemies.

You cannot do the job of parenting a preemie alone. You and your family need support. It's hard when you are going through the preemie experience and other folks are celebrating the full-term healthy births of their children. It can feel like you don't have the community you need around the birth of your child:

- Don't isolate yourself. I felt closed in a lot of times, and it's hard when you have to keep telling people the situation, but do just that. Tell people.

- Try finding social groups or support groups for parents with preemies. In the Resources section at the end of this book, I leave you contact information for some support services. Even when you have support, it can feel like you don't, because those who support you might not share the same experience. Find people who know the things you are going through because they have been through the same.

- Remember that everything is temporary. At the same time that it's a roller coaster with high highs and low lows, it's also a reminder that the lows, like your baby getting a blood transfusion, are temporary. Know that if your baby is jaundiced, it's temporary.

- Don't get too high on the highs or low on the lows. Try to stay grounded and stable so you are not anticipating the worst and getting anxious, or getting overly hopeful and getting anxious. Stay calm; every day is something new and you have no control, so try to keep yourself at a medium.

- Remember most of all that it's okay to not be okay and to reach out for community.

PART III

My God, My Faith

Sometimes all of the hustling and problem-solving in the world can't get you out of the paralyzing grief of death, disease, and heartbreak, but prayer and faith can see you through to a better place. Looking back, my mother's death took the ground from under me. What kept me from falling was the love of my faith community and my bishop. It's like they had been woven in place just before the bottom fell out.

When Dakota was born, prayer and my faith in God and community surrounded Dakota in the NICU, and that brought us through. Prayer messages on social media lifted us. "I'm praying for Dakota," "I'm praying for you and your family."

My experience with the miracles of a faith-based life that is so strongly rooted in the women in my family helps me to know, even today, that prayer and faith in God can heal me. Prayer and faith can heal my girls, and the generations of moms and daughters that have suffered through these same issues, and it gives us a safety net when all else fails.

7

A Family That Prays Together

The first time me and JR and Demi prayed together was the night Dakota was born. She had been whisked away from the NICU, and aside from seeing her beady ant eyes and slipping into a place of mortal grief, I hadn't seen her.

That first night, I was so sick and on so many drugs that I was high. I had forgotten about seeing Dakota's eyes when she came out of me. Everything was like in one of those dreams where you skip around in different realities. I somehow managed to sit my sick-self up in the bed and was trying to have a casual conversation with JR's teammates and their wives who came to visit me late after the game. They had all seen Dakota in the NICU, and I still hadn't really. I looked at them all tall and strong in their workout gear, and they looked at me with

IVs in both arms fighting infection but acting as if I was at the house entertaining like nothing had happened. I could feel their unsteady attention, afraid their words might make me crumble and turn to dust.

Looking back on it, I think a part of me didn't cross over from the two quick pushes. I was still in the moment of Kawana's and Ma's hands touching mine on either side of the bed, the living holding on to the almost dead. I think some part of me walked with death that afternoon.

Into that night I remember JR's tall shadow walking in and out of the room, going back and forth to see Dakota with his family. They reported back to me, but these were just words that floated above me. As the night went on and my brain started to feel solid again, not melted with fever, their words slowly had meaning. "She was born one pound. She lost a few ounces. She is intubated. She's gonna make it. She's gonna make it." All kinds of fake enthusiasm was in their voices. Her stats were all they really knew. I wanted out of that bed to go help my baby.

And then a woman dressed ready for the office, in a suit, came with papers, asking if JR and I wanted them to revive Dakota if they lost her. I knew what that meant. JR and I were both fully alert for that answer. "Come on now. She in here fighting! Don't ask us if we want to give up on her. Do what y'all have to do to keep her alive!" Some part of me was just repeating these words from holding on to my own mother. That feeling of sinking inside my chest while she shrunk away and other people were giving up on her. That shit wasn't going to repeat itself on me.

That's when I said, "Take me to see my baby." Sick as hell, I sat up. "Take me to see her."

They poked for a new vein, hooked my IV of fluids and antibiotics up on the pole of a wheelchair. JR lifted me from the bed to the chair and they wheeled me over to see Dakota.

JR, Demi, and I looked in the plastic case. Dakota's tiny arms and legs had little veinlike wires reaching for her, going into her, coming out of her, when she was only the size of Demi's hand. I was frozen in a type of shock and could feel JR looking at me and Demi looking at him. I had heard the words "premature birth," but I didn't know shit, didn't know what it looked like, didn't know the trauma of seeing your child like that, alive but her body not fully formed, skin like gel, not looking real. Like humans can't possibly be that small and be alive. I flashed to a childhood memory of my neighbor Mama Jessie in my East Orange apartment building showing me the newborn puppies in the bottom of her closet, and me seeing the hairless one and asking her, "Is that gonna be a puppy too?"

After a while of sitting there with my hand on the hard plastic of Dakota's incubator, hoping to feel her kick like when she was in my belly, I remembered how I used to sing to my mother and I thought, *Sing to her, Shirley.* I started singing the "ABC" song, which rolled into the Barney song, and Demi started singing with me. Then, I remembered praying with my mother and told myself, *Pray for her, Shirley.*

"Father God, please camp your angels around Dakota and carry her in your mighty hands. People are coming against her and saying she will not live, but we know with you all things are possible. If it be your will please allow my daughter to survive. In Jesus' name, Amen."

JR and Demi bowed their heads with me. JR's body was without sound but shook with tears. Our Demi was shell-shocked and confused. No child should ever have to stand in a moment seeing her parents falling at the force of a life-or-death struggle. She had been just like any little girl, saying mean things about her mommy bringing another little one in the world to take her attention away. I knew she was standing there thinking the words of her mouth had brought harm. JR and I held her hand, holding us in a circle, and I told her, "It's okay Demi. It's okay." We just stayed like that with me praying, *God, this is something we don't know. We don't know what to do, guide us.* I prayed until the storm of grief passed us into the next moment and I begged them, "Y'all please wheel me back to my room."

Those months in the NICU were a haven and a battleground for Dakota's life as she endured more surgeries that sometimes fortified her fragile body and other times further threatened her life.

Dakota was two weeks old. It was January 17, 2017. I was so excited when it appeared that Dakota was gaining weight, but in reality, Dakota looked larger because fluid was gathering on her brain from a peripherally inserted central catheter (PICC) line. The PICC line was the smallest available for preemies but was too large for Dakota's veins.

That morning, we met with the surgeon. It seemed like we walked through a maze of linoleum and doors and corridors forever before we got to the part of the hospital that didn't smell like antiseptic with the sounds of beeps and of carts being wheeled across the floor. This space was more like an office building with wooden doors, neat tables, and chairs inside. The surgeon was a six-foot-tall man who commanded the room like Pop as soon as he walked in with his stern voice. He brought us into a little conference room with a wooden table, black office chairs, and carpet. He held a laptop close and said, "Let's wait a few minutes for my colleague."

I did my usual courteous putting everybody at ease, even though that wasn't my job. "No problem. You know us, we don't have anywhere to go." He chuckled, but JR didn't. It was a serious moment; I just needed to keep it light because I couldn't stand to hear more bad news.

They told us that taking the old PICC line out and inserting a new PICC line was what was needed, but that required surgery, and since Dakota was fragile the way any baby bird is fragile, surgery might cause additional harm. They then said that without the medications the PICC line could provide, Dakota might die. I waited for more. I was thinking, *What the fuck are you telling us two separate awful scenarios for? You are supposed to be telling us what you are going to do about her having the wrong*

damn PICC line. It's not a solution to say you can fix it but either
way she might die.

I'm not a weak person. By that time, I had faced so many
life-threatening situations alone in my childhood and young
adulthood. "Weak" was not even part of my vocabulary. I had
survived abandonment and abusive relationships, but this was
beyond overwhelming.

I just said it. "So can you tell us what you are going to do?"

He cleared his throat, shut the little laptop, looked at his
colleague, and was like, "We actually have to ask you what you
would like to do, consent to surgery or enjoy the time you have
left with her."

Like a fucking magic trick, out came those damned consent
forms we were always signing, which were giving permission
to do some new measure or permission to leave her be so she
could stop suffering.

For somebody to be asking me if it's best to further threaten
my daughter's life or to hope for the best, which meant she
might die, was just too much. Who has to make those kinds of
decisions on the spur of the moment? And constantly? I didn't
even have a grasp of reality or time at that point, because the
new normal of the past two weeks of my life was a series of
constant life-changing shifts.

I remember sitting in my fuzzy sweatshirt and JR in his
workout gear. They left us alone in the conference room with a
big wooden table. JR and I sat there picking at the outlets in the
table rather than talking to each other. We knew the surgeon

was milling around in the hall, getting other shit done, but expected our decision soon. We looked at each other in that stunned way that we did when Dr. Young said she might need to take Dakota's unfinished little body from the harmful space of my body into the harmful space of the world.

I didn't know what to do. I just reached across for his hand. "Babe, what are we supposed to do? I don't even know. Everything is too quick."

He wasn't making eye contact anymore, and looked like somebody was pushing down on his shoulders when he said, "We said we was gonna keep doing what meant keeping her alive." I knew that was right, and let go of his hand for the box of Kleenex on the table. He sat back quiet while I let the tears and snot flow, then I took a deep breath. "Alright. Let's tell them to do the surgery."

We closed the blinds on the little window of the room, and I held JR's hands in mine and I prayed, prayed like I was in the pulpit. "Father God in Heaven. We know you are moving through us, know you are moving through our baby. We know your will is one of love and even when we don't understand that your will be done. We ask you to be with us today, to be with Dakota, to hold her in our family, to surround her with your love and to help us be strong as a couple, strong as her parents." JR and I were both sniffing then to keep it together, just exhausted. "Hold us in your light God."

Before these impossible days of life-or-death stress, I had stood in moments like this and prayed by myself. Some of my tears were because I was so grateful in that moment that I was not alone. JR and I had each other, and I had a faith community that I had sought out early in life. My cousin Danica drove our bishop, Barbara Glanton, seven hours from New Jersey to Ohio, and she just made it to the hospital to pray over Dakota with us before they took her to the OR. It was so important for our bishop to be there and pray over our Dakota, because if things didn't go the way we had prayed for them to go, we wanted her to be given back over to God.

Thankfully, she pulled through the surgery. So tiny, but so strong.

In the midst of the storm came a bright day. After thirty-four long days it was finally time, time for me to smell my Kota Bear, time for her to rest in my spirit and, most important, time for her to lay on my heart. She was two pounds and thirteen ounces when she received my first touch. This baby girl who didn't even have skin when she came into this world grew some skin on the nourishment of her family's love, on her community's literal food, on prayers that can't be measured. It was like a great big weight was lifted off of my and JR's chests and was replaced by the feather-light touch of this little brown angel. It was the blessing to let us know that no matter what came next, we could endure.

Me and JR and Demi got to hold Dakota's skin to our skin. I know one of the things that helped hold her in this life was getting to feel our expression of love through our touch.

I sang, "Like the dew in the morning gently rest upon my

heart." My happy tears instantly started flowing and the chills I got spoke volumes. Next in line was JR, also known as Poppa Bear. When I tell you this man was skinning and grinning, I'm not exaggerating. I felt his energy, it was so vibrant and contagious.

Dakota looked like a little shrimp lying on her dad's chest. I called my view of them a miraculous work of art because his tattoos surrounded her tiny body in such a unique way. She added another piece to the story that was already permanently written on his body.

When Demi got her turn, wasn't nobody going to tell her nothing. In the photographs from that day, she is holding her sister in her arms with that look on her face like, *Back up. She is mine.*

We all had grown to understand and comprehend that it is the little things in life that truly matter, the things you can learn from and appreciate, the experiences that help us grow, and this was definitely one of them. And that moment would carry us forward.

We received so much love and had so many people praying for us. The fact that we opened up and shared with the world, knowing we were not exempt from hardship, helped us immensely. People from all over the world were praying for Dakota, praying for our family, and I know that is what helped us to have some sense of normalcy while everything else was chaos. Sleepless nights, sometimes hungry because I was too stressed and exhausted to have an appetite, trying to keep the marriage afloat, trying to keep Demi sane and normal. Just chaos.

During those times, I would send my bishop pictures of Dakota. One day, she was at her church meeting with her leading pastor and others and they were all sitting around a table. She showed them Dakota's picture on her phone, and all of them reached in and placed a hand on Dakota through Bishop's cell phone to touch Dakota and agree and pray for her. I saw the video of this, and it warmed my heart. Everybody was standing in the gap for us in the way that I now stand in the gap for so many other families.

We were going to need that love to sustain us through the next 107 days of the roller-coaster ride. At the time, we could have never imagined all that was to come.

8

Custom-Fitting Faith for My Young Adult Years

I feel like my bishop has always been in my life, always part of my community of love. I have known her as a mother and grandmother in the community since I was five years old. I used to play with her granddaughter Quianna. But when I look back to see how I got to know the spiritual guide she is, I remember myself reaching to find something new at a brand-new time in my life.

Hillside, New Jersey, 2000
My sophomore year in high school, I was not afraid, or closed up, or soft-spoken like that little girl Lynette had found in the convenience store. Lynette and Kimberly and I moved to our

own apartment in Hillside near my mother's great-aunt Frances, the matriarch of the family. She was my grandmother Shirley's sister, the only person in our family at the time who had a whole house. I had family and friends, and Hillside was wonderful because it brought me even closer to my friends from Myrtle Avenue's Middle School who also went to Hillside High and closer to family. Aunt Frances, Uncle Danny, and my aunt Frances's daughter, my cousin Danica, lived upstairs, and my great-uncle John lived on the first floor. Danica was a little bit older than me but we went everywhere together.

One day, I was telling Danica how I didn't feel like going to our family's church, Bethlehem. We got to talking about how this just wasn't it, like wearing stockings and being one way on Sunday when we had music in our heads and dreams about who we wanted to be. It just wasn't us to remain in the house of worship that we grew out of. My childhood friend Quianna's grandmother, Barbara Glanton, was a bishop at a church in Newark, the Love of Jesus Family Church (LOJ). We were constantly invited, and decided to give it a try.

On the way there, we were passing by abandoned homes, all these crack fiends, and the police. It was in the hood! There were potholes in the street, panhandlers, and a guaranteed chance you might get a random police stop. I was like, "Danica, I'm not sure. This is in the *hood* hood." But we walked in and were hooked. It wasn't mega, but the perfect size to freely congregate and fellowship. Everything was purple to represent royalty: the chair cushions, the wall behind the pulpit, the stole draping the pulpit; purple was everywhere. There was a media area, where they played music through the speakers. It was like the nightclub of churches; they were playing gospel music with a two-step. We was like, "Hey, hey."

Women in there had on jeans, hoodies; and some had on their Sunday best; it was a great mix. At Bethlehem women had to wear dresses with stockings, and you didn't dare walk in there with pants on. The old folks at LOJ were more conservative, but you could wear whatever you wanted; they called it "come as you are."

Once we mingled with people, I found my spot boppin to the music. They played six or seven songs and had praise dancers, these teens my age who were doing Alvin Ailey–type modern dance to the songs. Music was near to my heart, and having that as the first part of the service was right for me. Then came the announcements, and then the bishop came to the mic and brought the house down with the Word.

Reverend Jackson from my other church, bless his soul, had that stern voice, but here, I was relating to everything Bishop said, because she was a Black woman. That day, I tapped into my spiritual side not worried about anything except for being me. My mother once said to me, "I would spend all my money to chase that first high that I would never feel again," but this was a good high to chase. Here, I got what I needed every time I showed up.

This was a big part of my sophomore year. I had my Bible and my notebook every time I went, and the Word was so on point, I couldn't take notes fast enough. And I never worried about going hungry, there was actual food there and food for my spirit. To this day, I still sit in the same spot, the back row to the left in front of the media sound booth, where the TV ministry records. When I turn around and look up, Danica is right there because she is in the music ministry now. I can't tell you how important it is that I just joined forces with Danica and decided to break camp from my main family church and find this new church home. Bishop ended up being there through every up and down with my struggle to keep my daughter healthy and to keep her in this life.

She was also there from the beginning. God put her in my path as a spiritual mother of sorts for a reason, because a couple of years after I started going to her church, the pillars of my new home started to crumble under all sorts of weight.

I was discovering myself as a young adult, about to launch off from high school out into the world. I was just happy and things were happening for me. I applied to Morgan State, was getting good grades, and prom that year was one of the happiest moments of my life. Lynette saw to it that I looked like a princess, and I felt like one too. I got my hair done and pinned up on my head, had the most beautiful burgundy formal dress, and even wore pearls. You couldn't tell me nothing. I had come a long way since that day Lynette saw a quiet little girl that she barely recognized in the convenience store looking malnourished with her hair all matted. I don't know how it's possible, but my smile turned into her smile, bright and happy. I guess if somebody looks at you like a mother, smiling for long enough, you take on the same smile. My mother wasn't there to see me off for prom, and I had gotten used to that. I couldn't predict when I might hear from her with a call that said, "Shirley, I'm getting myself clean," which just felt like a way to say, "I'm thinking about you" before she disappeared into the next high. But that day, I wish I had gotten a call so I could tell her the good news. I won prom queen.

Hillside, New Jersey, 2002

The next summer, I was preparing for my senior year, chilling with my family and friends. Aunt Frances had one of her usual cookouts. It was one of those times where everybody comes together. We might have been a family like any other with problems—this one not liking that one, this one out in the strcets—but we always came together for cookouts, and for some hard-core laughing and music. This time Tokunbo's father let him come. Every time I saw him, it was like time hadn't passed, because we were all each other had at one time, and we were the two who saw Mama at her worst. He just got a little taller every time, that's all. Not in a saggy diaper, but tall and chubby with still a little sag, but this time in his jeans.

It was unusual that his father let him come, because his dad was a little above us. He didn't know not to associate my mother's addiction with the whole family. Everybody was chilling in the backyard: cousins, aunts, and uncles. The grill was sending up that charcoal smoked-meat smell. Uncle Walter was the only person allowed on the grill because he knew how to "put it in the air," and his ribs are to die for. The music was playing Mary J's "Family Affair": "It's only gonna be about a matter of time, before ya get loose and start to lose ya mind. . . ." Danica was the dj for real, keeping the music going. Whenever my family got together it was always a damn good time.

I was dancing around in the backyard with my plate and Lynette got serious like PopaAuntie. "Come here Shirley. Sit down." She had her plate too and I sat on the back-porch steps next to her. "Shirley, I'm moving back to Irvington to an apartment there. I found a little two-bedroom place."

I was a year from graduating. I was about to tell her that I didn't want to leave my friends in Hillside to go back to Irvington High, but she was like, "Shirley, I'm not leaving you. Finish up at Hillside High and then we'll all be able to move back together."

By then she had Kimberly, Keyera, and Kalynn. There was no room for me anyway. I saw myself graduating and going on to Morgan State. I was feeling good, everything was all hopeful. I didn't want to feel left out, so I was like, "It's cool," and it was. I liked the idea of staying at Aunt Frances's with Danica and moving on from there. Lynette was a mother to me, but Irvington was close enough to Hillside. It would be good to just have a little bit of distance and try out my independence. I didn't let myself connect anything negative to my feelings back then, just happy-go-lucky Shirley.

When graduation rolled around, me and Danica were so

excited, because high school graduation wasn't accomplished a lot in our family. I was so happy, but things were kind of itching in the back of my head that I wished were different.

PopaAuntie, Lynette, aunts, uncles, and cousins were there. I was wearing white under my burgundy robe, white to mark a new beginning in my life. It was on a football field, that bright green against the royal look of all those burgundy robes, a really big deal. My mom wasn't there and at that point I wasn't tripping. I was thinking more about the sorrow that I would feel when I would soon be separated from my friends, and the joy of throwing my cap up, not like some character on TV, but me, Shirley. I actually felt my heart soaring around in my chest, feeling so damned good and so sad at the same time.

My high came down after the outfits and the lights were gone and we didn't have to get up and go to school the next day like the underclassmen who weren't finished with the school year yet. Everything just slowed down, and the excitement went away for me but stayed there for my friends. They were all going to universities and I was headed to Union County College. That was embarrassing. I had applied to Morgan State, but they lost my high school transcripts. I didn't feel it often, but in those days that slowed down after graduation and left me with no routine, or no place exciting to head off to, I felt embarrassed.

I wanted one of those parents who focuses on you, sits with you, and fills out all the paperwork and gets in people's shit if they lose your shit. I didn't feel like I had that; Lynette was a good guardian, but she also had her own kids to take care of. I didn't feel motherless often, but when I realized all my friends were leaving me and going to universities, and no one was pushing for me to get what I needed, it sank in. I just didn't feel like I mattered.

I tried to draw on my mother's voice like she was there. I remembered mostly the bad days, but I remembered my mother saying, "Shirley, don't ever do crack. You'll end up like this." I took that in as the motherly advice I needed. I knew that I wanted to stay in school and stay away from drugs and the streets. I told myself, *Shirley, be grateful County College is still college where you can take it to the next level.*

Problem was, I couldn't just stay up in Aunt Frances's house when her own daughter was dj'ing and becoming a successful entrepreneur, so eventually I called Lynette. "Can I come live with y'all?" Something in my pride didn't want to go back. I was a young adult. I didn't want go backward, but at the same time, I was really feeling lost. I needed home.

She had moved to an even bigger apartment with a first floor and a basement. She was still working in medical records and had a tight handle on her three daughters. I just wanted to be folded back up in that grounded reality. "Girl you know my home is your home." She was like, "Shirley you can have the basement and fix it up like your own apartment."

"That'll work." I breathed relief. I got a job at Mi Ohn Style hair salon on Chancellor Avenue in Newark and, with school, I got seriously busy. I didn't have time to fix up the whole basement, but I took one of the rooms down there and fixed it up like a little dorm room with my IKEA furniture, 2Pac posters, and my matching comforter and beige sheets. Yep, I got a big TV. Remembering my days with the mini TV and bed in the bottom of the closet, I had always envisioned having a big-screen TV, and I finally did.

I was determined and went to school every day. On Sunday me and Danica went to be in fellowship at LOJ. Nice people greeting you, and music, and good food. It was the highlight of my week. For two years, I kept up my routine with school, my job at the hair salon during the week, and church and family on the weekend. I knew the regimen in Lynette's house. I got up in the morning, got my turn in the shower, and was either in a cab, at that bus stop, or waiting for my ride from my boyfriend Lateef if I hadn't borrowed Danica's car. Things were going smoothly, and I was about to reach the associate's degree level. I knew that with determination and God's grace that I could go all the way and get my bachelor's degree.

Irvington, New Jersey, Fall 2005
One day, I was down in my little basement room studying with my glowing lava lamp lighting up the walls and my TV on BET in the background, and Lynette came down there and said, "Shirley, the phone is for you." I ran up the stairs thinking it was Lateef. It was my mother.

She sounded so weak. I remembered her voice and felt eight years old, like no time had passed. I got a knot in my chest and wanted to be near her. She said, "Shirley, I'm in rehab." I said, "Oh, Ma that's so good," but I had gotten calls like this before.

Darryl, Tokunbo, and I had that call so many times. We'd see our mother go to rehab then back to the streets, and had learned not to invest in any of that back-and-forth. But this time was different. I was more of a woman and knew I could mother her, or at least I thought I could. I thought I could tell God that I would take it from there and nurse my mother back from all the damage she had done to her body in my absence. I was about to start my junior year of college and I was going to do it all. School, handle things with my mother, everything that needed to be done.

I told Bishop Glanton, "My mother's trying to get clean. I know she can do it this time. She just needs people believing in her." We prayed on it and she found my mother a transitional house for getting clean in Brooklyn, Anchor House.

At first, my mother couldn't have visitors and we had to write letters to each other. She wrote me that she went to Great Adventure for the first time. "Shirley, I was so proud of myself. I had a little money on my card, and I got to spend it doing something fun. I can't wait until you can come visit and see what I got for you, a stuffed animal I named Jesus."

You know how it is when you are in love, feeling hopeful and looking at everything like the greatest wishes are going to come true, and everybody around you is seeing things for what they really are? Yeah, that's where I was.

Anchor House had monthly dinners for family members. The

aunts, cousins, and my brothers and I made shirts for going to the dinners, "Team Bertina." I was so happy that things were beginning to change.

Anchor House used to go around to sing at different churches. I went one time when Mama sang with them, and they were coming to Love of Jesus. I told the whole family and we packed the church. She was singing her lungs out. We were like, "Look at Birdie." She had on a green two-piece dress suit with gold trim and a jacket. They sang Donnie McClurkin's "I Call You Faithful." There's a part when he says, "Yes, yes, yes," and she was up there so happy. She was so little, and seeing her family there to support her, she was just beaming. It was one of her proudest moments and one of my proudest moments as her daughter. Every time I looked at her, I smiled.

The reality was that Mama was so frail, like a paper doll, paper thin, fragile. She kept saying, "Shirley you have never seen me clean. I want you to see me clean." I could see in her eyes all of this sorrow that I never saw before. I knew she meant it and that just made me more hopeful.

I went to school and did my classes, went to my second job at Branch Brook Park Roller Skating Center in Newark, and in the evening went to the Anchor House in Brooklyn. I hustled to mother my loved ones the way I learned from PopaAuntie and Lynette. I would come and spend time talking with my mother while playing in her hair. During this time, she was going through a great deal of emotions, and I sang and brought the light. My mother was getting clean.

One visit, she did that move that Lynette did at the barbecue. "Shirley come here." She had the photo album of the family that I made for her on her lap. "Come here." She patted her skeleton hand on the sheet, and for the first time, I saw what everybody else saw. My mother had a foot in the grave, but I shook it off and kept singing that R. Kelly mother-love song, "Sadie": "Early one Sunday morning, breakfast was on the table. . . ." She told me the truth, right while I was singing and turning the photo pages and letting her lean on me. "Shirley, I have lung cancer." I heard her, but I kept singing.

I told her, "That's why we gonna keep the recovery going and make sure you're eating right." I told her, "Your body is just weak and rebelling after the drugs. When we get your immune system on point, everything is going to be back on track."

Some part of me was along for the ride of her wish to get clean and to have her children experience the real Bertina Marie Harris. I needed that. There had to be some kind of way for God to work and make that happen. I told myself that the guilt and shame was the thing that made her stop, helped her have a rock bottom, and now she would get better.

I got into nurturing her the way I always wanted her to nurture me, and it was working. But I only know from looking back that I was in denial. My mother also had the AIDS virus.

When her T cells went up, she put on a little weight, and the virus became undetectable. I knew I was working that magic with God. But I was wearing myself out. I went to see my counselor at school and told her I needed to take a semester off because my mother needed me.

It was actually a beautiful time for us. I have always been the family historian, the one who collects and is always taking photographs. I got pictures from other relatives and brought them to her, and we filled up more photo albums. We sat and she told me who was who.

I looked in the mirror and I was the spitting image of her when she young. She must have been seeing that too, and said, "Stay in school Shirley. Don't be like me." She repeated, "I wanted my kids to see me clean." I just made a joke to keep it light. She sat there putting on that Noxzema that she just loved. She smeared it all over her face thinking she was doing something. I was like, "Chill out! You not Miss Clairol or L'Oréal."

That night, I told her, "I love you. I got you," before I put on the gospel CD that Danica made for her. I kept the weighted feeling in my chest from sinking, kissed her cheek, and made my way from Brooklyn all the way back to Irvington, New Jersey. I got to my basement room and fell out until the next day.

Then if it wasn't one thing it was another. My mother got blood clots in her legs; the cancer was getting worse. She had to get stents; she became frail again. The AIDS wasn't a factor, everything else was. Her body was being attacked from all of the days of walking the streets chasing a high with no food, no sleep, no one to protect her body from whoever might take advantage of it. I didn't know how I could stop it, but I tried.

Instead of going back to school the next semester like I told my counselor I would, I told my counselor, "My mom is sick. I still can't come back."

This was my first time completely quitting school. I started going to Brooklyn every day, where she was in the hospital.

In November, I made the executive decision to bring my mom home to Lynette's. I felt like I could love her back to health, feed her, take care of her, and everything was going to be like it should have always been—her as my mother, and me her daughter. She stayed with me in my room in the basement. I had her on the air mattress. I was in deep denial. She was so sick and frail. I was cleaning up when she couldn't control her bowels, running up and down the stairs trying to make her something to eat. I had to keep her hydrated. I stared at her when she slept to see if she was looking any better than the day before. I wasn't going to let her out of my sight the way I did when I was eight and she was just out there gone.

This time, she had tried to come back to me and I wanted to be there. One night, my mom said, "Shirley I can't do this," and we got her out of the basement where she didn't have any business being, and the family helped me put her in a nursing home in Irvington so that she would be nearby.

Aunt Anita, my mom's twin, came from Alabama, and we were around the clock, all the aunts, taking care of Mama. Bishop prayed, but we were told Mama would die in a week. I prayed to God, "Please don't take my Mama. Please help her get better." I didn't believe she was going to die even though she was unresponsive. One day, she got a little better and spent two months after that calling on everybody, especially me, Tokunbo, and Darryl, and told each of us that she was sorry for her addiction.

We sat her up, wheeled her in the shower. She was so fragile that the water hurt her body. It got to the point, for me, that I didn't want to see her like that anymore. I knew she was a hustler, a go-getter, because little memories seeped through, like her washing our clothes in the tub and wringing them dry, and now she couldn't wash her own face. That took a toll.

One spring morning, early 2006, I played her some music, one of Danica's new gospel mixed CDs. I paused the music and read the Bible to her, Isaiah 41:10, "Fear not, for I am with you . . ." Other family members visited, and the day went by, but I stayed with her. When I got too tired to stay awake, I was like, "Alright Mama. I'm getting ready to say, I love you. See you later." I had held in my head every day that I knew it was possible for her to get better. I knew God could heal and that it was possible. I was too tired to say that to myself that night. We only lived ten minutes from the nursing home. I got home and moved through the basement and into my little room. I was crawling-tired, got in my bed, and went fast to sleep.

Lynette woke me up an hour later and said, "Shirley, she is gone."

I just sat up in the dark. I didn't say anything. Lynette clicked on the light. I had been okay, in the dark, like still in my sleep, until she shed light, and I shed all my tears. She held me, because

Mama was her favorite aunt, and she had done what she could to hold on to me while I did everything I could to hold on to my mother.

I asked Lynette to leave me alone and I turned on my TV for comfort. Lil Wayne's "Hustler Musik" was on BET, and I zoned out. That steady beat, like my brain was just rocking like I was high or something. That song ain't but a few minutes long, but I felt like it played for hours. It had that melody where you felt yourself drowning in it.

That song means something to me to this day, like my first outlet after my mama died. I finally went upstairs with Lynette and sat on the couch. I put my big girl panties on. It was over, she was gone. I had to be her big girl and take care of her. With Lynette by my side, I did everything that needed to be done to arrange my mother's funeral.

I didn't hesitate. I knew to call on my bishop, Barbara Glanton, my other mother in spirit. She prayed with me and made it clear that for sure we would have the funeral at the Love of Jesus Family Church.

I didn't know as a young adult that I had laid a foundation of faith community that would sustain me through some of the most difficult times in my adult life. My faith helped me through the mostly bad days in the NICU and through to brighter days. I also didn't know at the time that I was about to go on a long roller-coaster ride in my adulthood of stuffing my emotions away and doing a superwoman routine that would last for years until God sent messengers to halt me and heal me.

No more tears, in that moment on the couch. I stuffed my emotions for the time being and hopped to it the way the women in my family had shown me to do. I wrote my mother's eulogy right then. "To know my mother was to love her. I am grateful for her life and she will truly be missed by us all. Bertina had a way to make you laugh so hard you would cry at the same time. She was the comedian in the family." Then I said, "Goodbye Mama."

Dropping Jewels

Keeping the Faith Through
the Valley of Shadows

A faith-based life has been linked to improved health outcomes for African American women, among those the capacity to endure poverty and weather the storm of a positive HIV diagnosis (Musgrave, Allen, and Allen, 2002).

That's no joke. So many times, life put what seemed like insurmountable obstacles in my path. But God continued to put the right person in place to keep me holding on in the worst of times. I don't know what I would have done without my cousin Lynette, without the ability to be with my mother at the end of her life and pray with her, without Bishop, who offered me so much guidance during the passing of my mother and the birth of my Dakota.

Each time, I got to the other side. My family and I weather the storms that come on a regular basis in life because that's life. But the calm is regular too. In those times I reflect on how much I have been gifted and I do the best I can to give that back. I become the ram in the bush for families with preemies struggling to figure it all out, and for other young women struggling to make it.

One of the things I like to tell women and young girls when I'm out there speaking about my experiences and offering hope is to build a spiritual practice so when the storms come, you'll have that to lean on. It doesn't have to be something fancy. For me it looks like:

- Checking in with my bishop and knowing that when I can't she will check on me.

- Going to a church or "getting in the house" even if you can't be at your own church.

- Praying. Prayer is powerful in your life and in the lives of those you are praying for. I know; nothing in my life has been by coincidence.

I have only prayed to one God my whole life, so there is only one source I pull from, Jesus Christ, the Holy Spirit, it's all intertwined. There are all religions and faiths to pull from. When you go from trauma to trauma in life you have to pull from something bigger than you because you are broken, and you can't pull from a broken place and expect to be strong enough to heal. So faith and me pulling from God has been a priority for me because it's been a method that I have used since I can remember learning how to pray. So allow your faith to be your clutch.

My God, My Faith

Everybody's faith practice doesn't look the same, just like when I was a teenager and I needed something different from the church my family had been attending. Find what is right for you, but do practice your faith, because our bodies are connected to our spirits. To keep the body healed and to maintain health we have to maintain our spiritual selves.

When things look like they can't get any worse, reach out to one of God's other children for a helping hand, and when you are blessed enough to hear God speak to you, obey his guidance. It may lead you to the fulfillment of your dreams.

PART IV

Therapy to Heal My Energizer Bunny

Women think they can do it all and just keep going, but we all hit a wall. My mother was nineteen years old when she had my brother Darryl, and then had me when she was twenty-three, and had my brother Tokunbo when she was thirty. She was a Black woman living off of public assistance in East Orange, New Jersey, with three kids at the time. The odds were against her. She was likely to hit a wall. The same is true of my cousin Lynette. She started taking care of me when she was a kid, and she kept doing so while raising her own kids. Her energy was gonna run out one day. And the same was true for me; I was a kid taking care of my brother and eventually my own mother and grew into an adult who struggled with issues of love, abandonment, and difficult pregnancies. So for me, a breakdown was gonna happen eventually, just a matter of time.

We convince ourselves that "We do what we have to do,"

because that's what our mothers and their mothers did. We are capable, yep, and capable of overwhelm and breakdown like every other human being. What we have to put into our generational understanding is that it doesn't mean we are weak if we ask for professional help. It's an extension of our strength.

9

One Year, Two Babies

On day 141 of Dakota's life in the NICU, my day started out relatively calm. I awoke to the sound of my alarm with the habitual mindset to get Demi up and ready for school. The pre-symptoms of a cold that she had the night before took hold, and my big girl did not feel well at all. I thought, *Of all days Demi is sick! Why today when her sister is due to come home?* I didn't let myself dwell on that negative thought. *No sweat, I'll just ask Auntie Anita to stay home and nurse Demi back to health while I make my way to the hospital.*

JR had to work so we agreed for him to meet me at the hospital. I still had a list of pointers I needed to ask the nurse while I waited for him to get there. Some of the things included picking up her prescriptions and learning how to properly give them to her, and learning the proper mix for her formula to put her on higher calories, as well as the oxygen and pulse monitor instructions. I was getting a little overwhelmed.

I felt the rush coming so I kindly asked Dakota's nurse to please ask everyone to give me some time alone to eat my breakfast and gather my thoughts before Grand Central Station opened up. Little did she know, I needed that time to shed some tears and thank God for how far he had brought Dakota. It was just a bittersweet day. For 141 days the NICU was our second home, it was my family of caretakers who offered me mommy guidance, and today that would change. So as I packed up Dakota's books I cried. As I packed up her clothes I cried. When I looked at her nurses I cried, and when JR walked into her room I cried. I was not just crying because I was leaving the familiar, I was going through various emotions and memories of the hard days that I needed to purge, to leave it all there.

After sniffing and snotting everywhere, it was time. Dakota's doctor still saved Dakota as the last preemie on her rounds. She wanted to save her for last because this was our last time getting Dakota's daily report. She told me "I signed for you to be admitted and I will sign for you to be discharged." With tears pouring like Niagara Falls they gave us Dakota's report for the day, proudly announcing her weight as five pounds and six ounces. "I now pronounce you discharged." And just like that, we got evicted.

There are no words in the dictionary that can describe JR's

and my feelings. I almost wanted someone to knock me upside the head with a frying pan, so I would know it was real.

On the drive home, we did not listen to any music. We were just silent, absorbing that this just happened. For the life of us, we could not find the words to describe our feelings or to even say anything on the ride home. He was driving and I was in the back seat snuggled next to the car seat, an image I had repeatedly dreamed that was now a reality.

When I first brought Dakota home I thought, *The struggle is over, we made it.* I had jumped over all the hurdles laid before me and life was, once again, supposed to be easier. Me and JR spent the first months trying to settle into life at home with a preemie. Needless to say, it got real real fast. JR and I became fully aware of all of Kota Bear's needs, and that our shit was going to need to be secondary to my daily life of learning how to properly care for Dakota at home—scheduling appointments and oxygen drop-off and pickup, all while managing a home, tending to my husband, and doing my best not to leave my pride and joy Demi behind. Yes, JR and I were still a special thing, but two parents with a daughter who required a special everyday life was our new thing.

It was like trying to find the rhythm to a new type of music you never heard before and your feet are going one way, your hands another. If I wasn't forgetting about a doctor's appointment for Demi, I was forgetting about a medication I was supposed to pick up for Dakota, and trying to figure out how to have food in the house for everybody to eat breakfast, lunch, and dinner, trying to remember to pay bills, meet with Demi's teachers for parents' day. *Oops, got to put gas in the car.* Got to, got to. And don't even mention sleep. My brain was just floating around in my skull during the day, trying to solve all of these puzzles on no rest.

Then on top of that, news interviews and JR's work life, and I was supposed to look all hair and nails and not look like my ass was about to bust out crying. But you know me, I did it all, the good wife who was at the game supporting my husband, the good mom who was at the school supporting one daughter, and at all the newborns' doctor's appointments supporting her preemie. I did it all with smiles and good attitude and jokes and making sure everybody was happy and taken care of. I did all the chaotic shit like it was some behind-the-scenes situation that needed to be handled.

A few months into this chaos, I found out I was pregnant with our third daughter, Denver.

All of a sudden, I was faced with all of the ways I had been living with the "go" button pressed. Nobody told me that mothering since I was eight years old, no older than my Demi, would catch up and knock my ass down one day.

It was my and JR's first anniversary. We had gotten married on my birthday, August 8, 2016. Mind you it had only been three months since we brought Dakota home. I had healed physically and she was in the clear for the most part. But emotionally, I still hadn't had time to process any of the past year of my life. JR and I went away to Mayakoba, Mexico, for our anniversary and were having a good time. Except I wasn't feeling like myself. The birth control pills were bringing about too much of a shift—I was getting hot and cold chills, some cramping, nausea, and night sweats. I told myself, *I need to switch back to an IUD or a Depo or something.* We got back from the trip, and things were on their regular roll. I transitioned two or three days back into being home and was at the basketball arena for one of JR's games. When you are a spouse they have special seating for you.

I saw my doctor and her husband and waved at them, and they came over and sat next to me in our section. I just brought it up, very direct like I always am. I told her, "Hey, I want to switch birth control."

She was like, "Sure, just take an at-home pregnancy test first and you're still going to have to take one in the office. That's standard for switching your birth control."

I was like, "Oh, that's no problem. I can go and do that in the bathroom right now." We laughed about it and I didn't think anything of it, just part of the routine for switching birth control.

I bought a test, and the thing showed positive. Dakota was only eight months old. I thought, this has to be wrong. So I made my appointment for new birth control. But you have to take the test in the doctor's office just to make sure you're not pregnant before they put you on something new. And lo and behold, I was having another baby.

I hopped into action. *Shirley, you ain't got time to be in shock. This is information you have early so you can prevent another difficult pregnancy.* I did my thing, stuffed the emotions and got to it.

It's never easy to move, but there I was with a nine-year-old and an eight-month-old with special medical needs, and JR in the middle of his season. He agreed that we needed to live closer to Cleveland Clinic's Hillcrest Hospital, where Dakota had received good preemie care. So we moved.

We were still getting through hurdles with Dakota, who wasn't even one year old yet. For a while I chose to keep certain things to myself, because I needed time without other people's reactions.

My doctor did know that I was pregnant again, and when I tell you that she was on my heels, she was all over me like white on rice about things I needed to do to ensure this pregnancy was as healthy as possible.

Eventually I swallowed the "pill" and digested the reality that we were having another baby. "Yay!"

It seemed like once I accepted the responsibility of being a new mother again, the weeks flew by. Everything was all good until January 2, 2018. I can remember so vividly, because it was Dakota's first birthday. I couldn't believe it; I had an appointment to get an ultrasound done on Dakota's actual birthday with all those memories of the day Ma rushed me to the hospital. I kept thinking, *How is it only a year later? My whole life has shifted.*

We still had family in town who came for the New Year's

party and to celebrate Dakota's first year of life, so I had my aunt and cousin join me at the doctor's office. I was told I would have to have a cervical cerclage done because my cervix was already beginning to open up. The tears immediately started streaming down my face while I was thinking, *Why can't I carry my babies full term?*

My doctor took a look and patted me on the knee for me to sit up. First thing she said was, "You have good instincts Mama!" She only knew from looking at my chart about Dakota's birth, but didn't know anything about the instincts I had been forced to mature into for the past year. She explained that my uterus was weak from my pregnancy with Dakota and still hadn't properly healed. She said that if I hadn't come in for an ultrasound on that very day, I would likely have delivered my baby early or have had a miscarriage.

They did the cervical cerclage to stitch up and fortify my uterus as an outpatient procedure, right then and there. Then my doctor said something that is hard for an Energizer bunny to pull off. "Shirley, you are going to have to be on bed rest." I started crying again. I was like, *Damn, why can't I carry my babies? I got to get stitched up, I got to be on bed rest.* It was a whole additional experience for my body and mind, on top of the pregnancy and having an infant at home.

For some reason, women feel like it's a sin and a shame to tell anybody that we are tired after we have had our babies. It doesn't mean you aren't the most grateful overjoyed person to have received the gift of life. It means your body either turned itself inside out or somebody turned your body inside out and you are supposed to recover from that. But the baby has arrived, so rather than recover, you have to hop to it.

It means in the case of women with preemies that right after having your body turned inside out you begin dealing with the trauma of the life and possible death of your own child. The mind and the body under the best of circumstances go through war to bring this gift of life, and then everybody looks at you like, *Chop chop. Time to show you can feed, diaper, and nurture,* when you haven't even put yourself back together yet. Then if you have more than one child . . . I can't even finish that sentence. Where did I even get the mentality that I can just do whatever needs to be done no matter what? Where do any of us get that mentality from?

It's because we live in a society that can block the path at every turn at getting a better education, getting the resources to support our children, finding the love that we are worthy of. Being in survival mode to duck and dodge and strategize to get basic needs met can make anybody feel like they can do anything as long as it takes, with undying endurance. But that's a myth, Black women aren't machines. We wear out and, eventually, all that fight catches up with us.

10

Doing What You Have to Do

As a young woman, I had to get shit done or get caught without a place to live, or without a job. I learned a long time ago to be on the hustle at all times, but I never learned to turn it off.

After my mother passed, I don't know where I got the strength and courage and the ability to be able to do everything. In the aftermath of the pain, I was the Energizer bunny. I had to approve her dress and her makeup. I took her clothes to the funeral home, her favorite church outfit, that green two-piece dress suit with gold trim and jacket that she wore to sing with her rehab choir. They put her hair in a little Afro because it started falling out real bad from the cancer. It was a quick turnaround, not dragging it out two weeks waiting for people to come from down South.

I was so happy about all the people who came. My siblings and close family members were in the front row. My girlfriends and coworkers from the hair shop were there too. People from the rehab in Brooklyn were there. It was an outpouring of love. She was loved by so many people.

I had a smile on my face, like I was entertaining folks at a party. I was strangely happy because I had seen her suffer my whole life, and now she was free. I stood up strong and proud of who she had become in the year that she was clean. I got to see all of it. I saw her live, and become healed, and lose her health all over again. I was happy that she was free from not being able to wipe her own ass. That's what gave me strength, and it would have broken anybody else down to puzzle pieces.

I sat down in the front row next to Tokunbo and Darryl. Everybody said their word or two about what Mom meant to them, and I just kept smiling, because I was happy knowing that her spirit could hear all of that praise. When everybody had said what they wanted to say Bishop Glanton spoke the Word and it was time for the processional, when everybody walks up with the music playing and goes to the casket to touch her hand, take a last look and say goodbye, then come back around to the immediate family for hugs or condolences.

I sat there with my brothers, smiling and ready to do my part of shaking people's hands or giving them a hug. The song that played next was "Yes" by Shekinah Glory Ministry. It stirred the memory and the emotions I felt that day when my mother stood in the place where she now lay. Her choir singing, "My soul says yes. Yes, yes, yes."

Family and friends went up to the casket and walked back to greet me, and I was ready to console them instead of them consoling me, but I just kept hearing "Yes, yes, yes," and seeing Mom so happy singing with her mouth wide open and, out of nowhere, I broke down, screaming. I leaned back and everything that I had in my soul eternally, everything I had been strong about since I was a little girl and strong about for everybody else, even in that situation, just broke. I wailed from my gut to the ceiling of the church, to Heaven, to God.

I screamed and screamed and screamed, and it was a ripple effect. My brother Tokunbo started hollering, then Darryl broke down. PopaAuntie and Lynette tried to console me, but for those few minutes, I was gone. It was as if all of my emotions hit me all at once in that moment.

I was weak and out of it after that. Spent, empty, as if I had left my body. Everything was gone. I don't remember anything that came after that moment at Mama's funeral.

My mom died at forty-four. She didn't even get to live a young woman's life. Only clean one year. I felt robbed, not just for myself, but also for my younger brother. I felt lost. *Where do I pick up now?* For the first few weeks, I was in a daze, going to work at the hair salon, coming home to Lynette's basement, just numb with hurt and confusion, wondering what happened.

One day I was resting after work and Lynette came to the

basement. "Shirley we need to have a conversation. I'm going to move down South. I'll make sure you are set up when the time comes." I was half-asleep. So I didn't feel that I had just been hit in the head. I was like, "That's cool. That's cool. You know me. I'm gonna stay here. Go back to school." I fell back to sleep only half-understanding.

The next morning before light, I was just snoozing away, and I heard hustling and bustling over my head. I heard Lynette's footsteps coming down in the basement and I looked at my alarm. It was three a.m. "Shirley, we gonna leave and go down South now. You good to stay here another month."

"What?" I was half-asleep and couldn't make too much sense out of what was happening. I just said, "Okay," trying to be nice. I went back to sleep again and woke up a few hours later. I went upstairs and it was empty, no table, no bed, no couch. Them niggas wiped it clean. I was by myself. I just had my room and a toilet. I had no money. I was working at the hair shop and all of my money was for helping with the bills. I was like, *Them niggas left for real.*

I was in shock. I went back downstairs and lay down and woke up at eight a.m. because someone was ringing the doorbell. I went up the stairs, and I heard somebody walking through the house. I was scared, about to shit my pants. I opened the door from the basement into the apartment and it was the landlord, who was this African man. He said, all mean, "Where is your mom?"

I said, "She left a couple of hours ago to go down South. She didn't tell you?"

He said, raising his voice and waving his hand, "Your mom is backed up on the rent, ducking my calls." He had been hustled by my cousin.

I said, "I'm good to be here though right? Because she said that."

He looked at me like I was crazy. "No! You have until noon."

He turned around all matter-of-fact. "I'll be back at noon to padlock it." He thought Lynette was my mother, so did I, and he took everything out on me that had transpired between them.

I was like, *Shirley, do what you got to do.* You know how we do, just pick up and roll on when life gets rough.

I called Lateef, the guy I was dating. The hustle was on. He used his truck and I took my clothes and left my IKEA bedroom furniture because there wasn't any time for all that. Quianna's mother offered to let me stay with her. She had extra space because Quianna was away at college. So I stayed there in the attic.

The period from 2005 through 2006 was definitely the year of being required to do so much that I didn't even have time to deal with my feelings. I just knew I had to do what I had to do, and the automatic survival button was in the on position.

So many of us go through the pileup of birth, death, job loss, home loss, major life hurdles with no time to do anything but be in superwoman mode, and our emotions get bottled up and start to make us sick. When Mama died and Lynette moved, I remember people saying, "Don't hold it in, don't hold it in." I don't know what I was supposed to do with it. I had to live, make money, pay bills, have fun, just like any other twenty-one-year-old Black girl.

I gave it to God, but that didn't keep it all from settling into my blood, didn't keep me from reaching for and wanting things to be good with family. That's all I wanted, family, and to follow what Mama said about staying away from the streets and making something of myself. So right then and there, I started holding on and holding up as a grown-ass woman, because I thought that's what grown-ass women do. But life doesn't stop throwing you curveballs. How much holding on and holding up is a woman supposed to do?

11

Postpartum Times Two

In February 2018, I finally had to quit running here and there. The doctor told me "bed rest" in January and in order to carry Denver to full term, it was time to sit my Energizer bunny butt down. I didn't have a choice; in addition to the cervical cerclage, I had the same life-threatening group beta strep infection that flared up during Dakota's birth. So I'm in the bed, getting weekly antibiotic shots in my buttocks, while taking care of my nine-year-old and my preemie. I couldn't have sex. I was on two different vaginal medications that JR had to put up in there every night for me. Where was my womanhood, my body? History seemed like it was repeating itself with more force. It was like I had gone back into battle when my wounds from the previous battle had not yet healed.

I'll spare y'all the months of watching way too much reality TV, way too much yelling at JR and Demi, and way too many nights trying to sing Dakota to sleep. Luckily, our next baby was carried to term and came into the world a healthy girl. JR and I named her Denver after the city where our love first took root and blossomed.

I was blessed, but I was lost. Think about the short timeline from sitting around on New Year's Eve only four months pregnant, shooting the breeze, to a year and half later. I had two infants and a preteen, and my body had been through hell. It's like I went outside of a door where there was nothing on the other side, and the door shut behind me. But y'all know how it is, the world of things that got to get done just kept on spinning whether I came along for the ride or not.

I was raised to believe I was capable of cooking three meals a day, cleaning, being strong, and getting it done. So that's what I did, until I was "doing" without stopping to assess the wear on my mind and body over the year. Self-care wasn't something I had modeled for me. The women in my family just "did" until the day when they couldn't "do" anymore. And all that doing was catching up with me.

I was yelling at everybody all the time. I didn't have tolerance for anything or anybody and had two crying babies. Poor Demi was doing the best she could to help out. She had followed in her mother's footsteps and was a good big sister to her siblings. But still, things began to topple. JR had to be on the road, so I didn't have him right there as my emotional rock, somebody to vent to. That's when I started accusing him of having an affair.

Denver was about to turn one. Dakota was a year and a half. JR told me to reach out for help. I remember it was summertime. And I won't forget that JR had just won the Championship with the Eastern finals. After all of that, he just wanted to spend some time with the fellas and go to Vegas. He went. Me being the emotional being that I was at the time, and the postpartum depression setting in double with the two babies, I started calling him and harassing him. I accused him of all sorts of foolishness and affairs. "You just want to go out there and be with somebody else. You want to leave me here with these two babies."

At the end of the day it was very selfish on my part because he had told me, "Let's start reaching out for help." He had seen everything I was going through in the house with the girls and he would do what he could, but a mother is a mother and the kids are going to keep reaching for her. The reality that he kept telling me to get help and I wouldn't stands out in my mind, in retrospect, along with the pressure of being a new homeowner.

We had just purchased a house in New Jersey. So another move with babies and a preteen. "There's money babe. Hire someone to help." But the help I needed was more than just logistical. Things weren't right in my mind. In my head there was just the pileup and him wanting to go away.

I made it an unpleasant getaway weekend for him. I was calling, accusing, nagging, texting unpleasant messages, nitpicking. I wouldn't let it go long enough for him to enjoy himself, all because I was unhappy with myself.

I was depressed, which wasn't a thing anybody in my family grew up talking about. I had feelings I didn't know what to do with. So I projected it all onto him, rather than saying, *Shirley you need help. Hire somebody or something.* But it was easier to blame him. He came back at me saying, "I'm not doing anything wrong! When I get back, we have to talk, because you not acting like yourself." He noticed it in me, and I started to notice it as well. That's when I began to realize things weren't right, and I was starting to spiral and started asking myself, *What's wrong Shirley? What's wrong?* I was hitting the wall.

There's been times in my and JR's lives and in our marriage where yes, it was him making things how they were and causing issues, but this time, it was me. I just wasn't willing to get help even though I was falling apart.

Then my body just said no more. One day, I was up, changing diapers, trying to make sure Demi got on the bus, zooming around like a robot, and my sciatic nerve, the single largest nerve in the body, spoke up. I just buckled at the knees and that was that. I couldn't do anything even if I wanted to. I was forced to call on my cousin and my niece for help with changing diapers. When they left every day, I kept insisting I could handle it from there with Demi's help.

Therapy to Heal My Energizer Bunny

I was still holding up the exterior of the beautiful wife of an NBA All-Star—hair and makeup on point. I was continuing the work I wanted to do for other mothers with preemies. I was packing boxes for UPS to make sure other moms could have baby-monitor cameras in the NICU. This part was helping to keep my mind and heart happy. But my body just kept screaming, *Sit your ass down!*

Both Dakota and Denver survived difficult pregnancies, that was a blessing. But now I was fighting for my mental health.

Pain talks to us, to let us know we are not invincible. The stresses of another difficult pregnancy, the lack of recovery time from Dakota's birth, and a lifetime pileup of stressors rained down on me. And that was the start of a downward spiral. You know how sometimes you are long past the moment of falling apart, but you keep moving and doing, so you never even feel anything? I was laid up in back pain trying to manage my house from the bed and found myself sliding full speed downhill into depression, unable to function or ask for help. Eventually I had to hire somebody to help me with the kids because, like it or not, I was in so much pain in my body and in my mind, I couldn't move. Thank God for modern medicine. But medication and the chiropractor were temporary fixes that set the Energizer bunny back in motion.

It was the end of summer, and our regular schedule was for us to leave New Jersey and return to Ohio for JR to get ready for training camp. His little break was about to end. Time to move again: pack the girls' lives back up, hustle back to Ohio, more mommy stress.

When we first got to Ohio we had to stay in a hotel, because our lease at our previous home there had expired. Me in the hotel with the preteen and the babies, it was a lot. I was so unhappy. That's what I mostly remember, because with that kind of depression the memory gets foggy too. We finally found a townhouse, and as the wife it was my job to get it situated and decorated. All of this should have been the good stuff. I should have hired the help I needed with the kids, but I was raised to be a strong Black girl and now a strong Black woman.

I was walking around with the same mentality that I have to do everything. I was finally in a situation where the financial freedom was there. I had the ability to pick up the phone and hire whoever I wanted. But I just did not do it, and it caused me to be in a situation where I was drowning, unable to keep my head above water for any decent amount of time.

Sometimes when we can't call for help, God sends a messenger to call us. I was in the townhouse, sitting on the bed. I had Denver in my arms and I was crying, just crying and crying beyond a thought of even knowing which thing I was crying about, and the phone rang. I saw it was Bishop Glanton, but I didn't answer while I was crying. Something told me to pick up the phone, tears and snot and all, and call her back. I did, and I told her the truth as best I could.

Therapy to Heal My Energizer Bunny

"Bishop I don't know what is happening to me. I had the babies back to back. I feel like I'm spiraling out of control. I don't even want to be bothered with my children. I don't know what to do. I'm overwhelmed physically and emotionally, and I'm losing my way."

She calmly said, "Shirley, have you ever talked to somebody professional?"

I was like, "No."

She said, "I have a therapist to refer you to. He does marital counseling and individual counseling. So you can take into discretion what you and JR need or what you need individually and give him a call."

I was feeling better just talking to her and hearing that there was something I could do about my situation. I said, "Okay Bishop," and I took the number and hung up.

I didn't waste any time, because I couldn't imagine my situation getting any worse than it already was. I really felt like I needed something to save my life. I picked up the phone and called. The therapist was in New Jersey and he said we could talk over the phone, or I could fly home depending on what I felt my needs were right then. I knew that I was in such a broken place that I needed to sit in front of his face in his office. I got on a plane and flew out to see him.

That is my therapist to this very day. I had to make myself vulnerable and reach for help and that was the end of the Energizer bunny and the beginning of healing.

The clouds slowly, slowly started to clear. And God dropped even more things in my path to help me. These opportunities were always there, but I was spinning in the chaos and couldn't see them.

In January 2019, my best friend, Kawana, who was also going through it, got in touch with me about a retreat called Sedona Soul in Arizona. A retreat? I did something I had never done but needed to be done a long time ago: I went on a retreat.

Dropping Jewels

How to Turn Off the Energizer Bunny and Get Help

Postpartum depression is the real deal. I felt it all unraveling even though something in me kept saying, *You don't get to fall apart Shirley.* Something else was saying, *Woman you should have fallen apart years ago.*

Studies have shown that African American women who grew up in poor financial and social circumstances are more likely to experience postpartum depression, but these studies also show that seeking therapeutic support and going to support groups are what can help us realize we are not alone and we are capable of surviving this time of deep depression (Broomfield, 2014).

As Black women, we are taught to keep everything bottled in and bottled up. We don't realize the stressors this places on our bodies, on our minds, and on our emotions when we carry around all this trauma from childhood to adolescence to adulthood. A lot of this we put on ourselves because we don't feel like it's okay to speak up or that people are listening to us when we say "Ouch" or "I need help!" We get scared that they are going to think we are weak and that they will then do what society does to Black women, take advantage of us.

Imagine (and most of you won't have to) growing up without your father, and your mother is absent because she is addicted to a substance. Imagine you have lived through molestation and a host of other things in your life and you have no outlet. It's like bricks are piling up on your body and they get heavier and heavier when you never even built up a solid foundation.

Yes, breathe on that word.

Then on top of that you insist on living a life where you can do everything in order to make everything in your life, and in everybody else's life, better. We constantly put out and don't take in anywhere near as much. It's just not a sustainable reality.

Trauma is trauma, stress is stress, hurt is hurt—major or minor, race related, or life related. Postpartum depression doesn't know your race. It doesn't say, *Ah, damn, you already been through a lifetime of shit, then let me skip over you*. It's a biological thing that happens with your hormones, and if you add a lifetime of Energizer bunny bottled-up stress to that, it's a Molotov cocktail.

Get help!

That's the advice I want to offer you all, even if you are estranged from your family or friends and don't have that backup. You need people, you need support.

Therapy to Heal My Energizer Bunny

- Do not isolate yourself. When I was in the situation of my postpartum depression, I felt closed in. Even sometimes when you have support, you don't feel supported because your friends and family want to keep asking you questions that you don't have the energy to answer. For instance, your family might not know what to do. "Can you tell me what I can do Shirley?" They are trying, but they don't know that you don't have the energy to tell them how to help you. If you did, you'd just help yourself. When this happens, don't isolate. Say, "Just be here," and guess what? They will be there, will see you losing your shit, and will figure out how to help.

- Seek support groups. These are people who have gone through the same thing. If you can't find one, make your own by blogging the way I did.

- Go to therapy! This might be most important. Therapy is okay. You need to be heard. You might have been taught to take it all to God, and pray, pray, pray. But we are in real times. I need a real person to act as an extension of God's communication to me. Check out the Resources section of this book for some links for your mental wellness.

- And it is also okay to put your daughters in therapy. That was foreign to us, but they can benefit from what we now know.

- Read about healing and about your body and its systems and about what you need to be mentally and physically healthy. Most of us live our whole lives with no information except the memories of the trauma and abuse and the recycling of generational curses. You need some new information to be thrown in to disrupt that recycling so that you can make something new for yourself and your kids.

PART V

Peeling Back the Layers

Admitting I was not superwoman, and reaching out for mental wellness help, was the beginning of me falling apart and evaluating my life so I could put it back together as the healthy version of me. It was the beginning of my healing. I'm not saying drop God and pick up therapy. I'm saying your faith practice and your mental health practice go hand in hand.

God is in communication with me always, but I am here in the flesh and need somebody to sit down in front of me in the flesh and say, "Listen, up is up and down is down." You know, I need a real-life reality check to offer me guidance to keep me from losing it and to help me to unravel everything that is beyond my solo understanding of things. Someone to help guide me so I don't explode with this buildup of stress in my Black-woman body, mind, and emotions. After the day I called a therapist, every step I took lit up my new life in front of me and helped me to find more tools for my healing.

I am saying this to everybody reading this book. You have to go backward to go forward. You have to figure out what the bricks that are piled on your chest are made of. You have to investigate your past to find out what is causing your Energizer bunny behavior, your people-pleasing chaos, your superwoman act, in order to be able to make healthier choices.

It can be hard to dive into your own stuff to figure yourself out, but being in therapy, reading self-help books, and being in support groups helped me to see the most important thing. The love I was driving myself crazy looking for was within my everyday reach, my children. If I didn't take the journey into my shit, I would have repeated the cycles.

My first step was to get vulnerable with myself:

Who am I? I am a woman who sometimes don't know who she is. I am a woman who does not know what normal is. I am a woman who has abandonment issues, trust issues, a lack of self-worth, and other inequities. I learned life the best way I knew how. I do all that I do from the kindness of my heart. But when it is not good enough it hurts because I am truly giving my best. I am worthy of being taken care of, but I need to take care of me so people can see it.

Sometimes I don't know how to take care of me. What does taking care of Shirley look like? I am always afraid that someone will eventually leave me because I am so used to being left.

It is easier for me to believe in everyone else and not myself; sad but very true. I have issues and I do need help. I often feel worthless, because I measure my worth based on how people treat me versus how I treat myself.

I have a hard time letting my children loose because I would never want them to feel like, Mommy left me, because that's what was done to me. I want to truly move beyond my past and heal. Every time I believe I take a positive leap forward, I am knocked back down, by people's words, triggers, and actions. It's almost like being told no matter what you do, you're not good enough. Or, I'm always made to feel like I'm always fucking up. Which causes me to shut down on so many levels.

I am speaking my truth, because I base my well-being on others being well, and I believe speaking and writing my truth is good for us all.

12

Girl Meets Boy

I know a lot of folks make the connection between looking for a mate and their relationship with their fathers early in life, but I only recently, here in my thirties, showed up to this reality. There was no getting around it. In therapy I had to face my daddy issues. I certainly can't pass on to my daughters a healthy understanding of men and relationships unless I take a hellishly good look at that daddy/boyfriend parallel.

Newark, New Jersey, Spring 2007
The spring after my mother passed away, I started down the right track with some self-love. I got a place of my own in Newark. I was proud of myself working at the hair salon and at

Branch Brook Park Roller Skating Center. It was about time I had my own place, where I could make things the way I wanted them to be. I was on the second floor of a three-family house on Goldsmith Avenue. I had a living room, and a little room for a bed and a TV for my brother when he started living with me. To the right was the dining area, but I made it into my office. There was a little hallway, then the kitchen, a little bedroom to the left and one to the right. It was the perfect size for me and my oldest brother, Darryl. We had a spot. We were grateful. It was a huge step up for it being my first apartment. I was like, *Okay Shirley you got a two-and-a-half bedroom in the Weequahic section of Newark.* The apartments were big over there, not little studios or basements. I was moving on up like George and Weezy.

It was May and nice out. I invited everybody; family by day for just the housewarming part and friends and homies at night to both celebrate and watch the fight that was coming on TV. I had to go food shopping, clean house, couldn't even get dressed, all day cleaning from ceiling to floor. The place smelled like some serious Mr. Clean and I had the windows open to catch that fresh breeze.

You know how I do; I love to entertain, so there was a vibe. I was boppin around to music making sure everybody had some Popeyes chicken, some rolls, greens, and was comfortable with drinks in their hands.

A mutual friend, Jamar, called. "I want to bring my friend

JR. Is it cool?" I didn't think nothing of it, I'm a people person, always love for whoever.

I said, "No prob at all bro."

When JR got there I greeted him like everybody else. He was tall with fair skin and a meek half-smile. He had on a fitted cap, oversize white T-shirt with some baggy jeans, and white Air Force 1 sneakers. I made sure he had a place to sit. He sat down in my kitchen to a plate of Popeyes chicken. I got him a drink, told him, "Make yourself comfortable. Make yourself at home," and I kept it moving. I was busy making sure everybody had a good time.

As the day progressed, food transitioned to game snacks. I mixed and mingled, even while everybody was staring at the TV, and passed him and was like, "You okay, you need any-thing?" He was cool, sitting off to the side, conversating with his homeboy Jamar.

He stayed a few hours. I didn't have much of a conversation with him, because I was so busy entertaining. One hundred per-cent, I don't remember knowing that he was in the NBA and didn't care at the time. That was our first encounter.

Jamar called me a day or so later and asked if JR could have my number. I didn't really want to release my number to him because I briefly heard at the party that JR was dealing with another friend of mine. Apparently, they were just talking, not in a girlfriend-and-boyfriend thing. Lateef and I had gone our separate ways months earlier, but I was also dating a little bit on and off myself. Mostly, I was working my two jobs and making a good place for me and Darryl, and by then Tokunbo too. Eventually I told Jamar that he could give JR my number. I figured there wouldn't be any harm in that.

He called me from time to time and told me his new number whenever he changed numbers even though I barely used the old one. I would be like, "Oh, how you? Great, thanks. Good to hear from you," and I kept it moving. I was healing from losing my mother, and I was working to find my grown-up life. What I didn't know was that summer, JR suffered a major loss that would change the course of his life. He ran a red light one night with his best friend in the car, resulting in a major accident. JR walked away from the crash; his best friend died. But that was in the background. When two people come together, there's a trail of shit a mile long that they both bring. We was both walking around with loss, which I can say now was part of the attraction in ways that we weren't aware of at the time.

At the end of the summer, Jamar got married to my childhood friend Quianna. JR and I ended up groomsman and bridesmaid. It was August 2007. Only a little more than a year had passed since my mother died and only two months had passed since the death of his best friend. The wedding was held in Maplewood at Quianna's aunt and uncle's house and the reception was in the hot backyard.

That Usher and R. Kelly song was playing, "Same Girl." Another guy was dancing with me and JR came sauntering over. The wedding was the first time we'd seen each other since my housewarming party. He and my friend put me in a sandwich and kept dancing. It was all still laughter, and the song was all sexy blaring, "We messing? With the same girl," but I was like, "Hold up. Get me up out of this like y'all actin like I'm some ho."

Then JR and I were dancing one-on-one, and he whispered all head tilted like talkin game, "Are you gonna give me a chance?"

I told him, "I don't know. You used to talk to my girl, and I have two jobs, and I'm enjoying my life right now." And that was that for the moment.

He kept calling me, though. He asked me several times to come to Denver where he was playing for the Denver Nuggets. Around Thanksgiving, I finally went out there for a weekend and that was all she wrote.

On the flight, in my head I kept doubting, thinking about the whole NBA thing. *I don't have time for being all in the scene of niggas acting Hollywood.* Somewhere in my head I was probably also thinking, *Is he just gonna have me go through all this and leave me?* I got there and it was nothing like I thought. I got to see who this boy was, contrary to my assumptions. It was magical. For him it was like a shock that I wasn't hung up on the NBA. I was like, "You are a person like me, just a different occupation."

We sat on the couch and shot the breeze: binge-watched *Martin* and *Die Hard* movies, ate ice cream. Then like best friends we got out and went bowling. I didn't feel like I had boundaries,

I felt like he was a guy from around the block who I knew all of my life, not all Hollywood. The best thing is that we laughed our asses off. I cooked and cleaned, like the shit was relaxed and domestic right off the bat. He made me feel like it was about me. Things were so comfortable that weekend that the lovemaking came as natural as everything else.

After that weekend with him we made it official and I got tattooed, on my wrist, his signature along with our starting date, November 11, 2007. Looking back, I wouldn't advise my daughter to date a man for a few weeks and get his name tattooed on her body, but hey, that's where I was at. Rick Ross said it best, "She in love with a G so she tatted my name."

Those beginning phases of our lives included a lot of traveling back and forth between Colorado and New Jersey, which is where we both called home. I looked forward to going to Denver, but always looked forward to getting back to my work at the hair salon and the skating rink and working with my brothers to keep up our apartment. It was my life. But I was always trying to see if JR was going to be playing a game in Philly, New York, or New Jersey so we could keep it close to home. It was full and exciting to be in love with him and also with the life I had built for myself.

I know those weeks of falling in love left a positive mark on our hearts that keeps us fighting for our love today. When there were no kids, no extra bitches, no pride, just us. Those days set the tone of our love.

A month later, Christmas 2007, I was back home in my

apartment on Goldsmith. I was on the phone with my aunt Kathy, the youngest of my mother's sisters. I was about to go back to JR's house when she just said something slick: "You know Erics ain't your real father." Erics was the man who came and went from the picture. I called him Daddy because I didn't know any different.

I was like, "Then who is?"

She said, "Gary."

"Who the hell is Gary?"

My mom was deceased, and I couldn't ask questions. I called JR who was in New Jersey at the time, and I told him I was just on the phone and found all this out. I was questioning out loud, "What is this all about?"

JR tried to console me with his sleepy deep voice, "Don't worry about it babe. Don't worry." In retrospect, here I was a few weeks fresh in a relationship and already coming to my man with the bullshit. He must have been thinking, *Wait, she ain't got no father present. Who she thought was her father ain't her father.* . . . I didn't know it at the time, but I was taking it to him first hoping he would just soothe that daddy-loss and fill in.

I went back to his place in Colorado, where we set up a life that was domestic and everything just flowed, him on the road a lot, me at home making things nice for us. I put my daddy concerns away so I could try to just enjoy the life God had blessed me with. When I look at it now, I see that I was making decisions and moving around with my daddy concerns in tow the whole time. They say trouble don't last always, but they forget to tell you that sometimes trouble from every area of your life can flare up at the same time, like roads that all cross in one jumbled-up traffic jam.

In 2009 the happy roads and the hellish roads in my and JR's lives met up. I found out I was pregnant. We were so excited. I was twenty-five years old, about to have my first baby, the same age my mother was when she had me. We said if it's a girl, we will call her Demi, because we both liked "D" names for girls, and it would be easy on a job application—Demi, not something like Deminiqua. If it was a boy that would be a no-brainer: Earl Smith Jr. III. We would keep the male line of his family going.

That's when all of the questions of being the daughter of a man I didn't know started tapping on my shoulder again. It wasn't long before we found out we were having a girl. I needed to know who I was so I could explain to my firstborn who she was. Like, I was getting freckles. I was in the car looking in the vanity mirror. *Will my baby have freckles? My mom didn't have them. Where were these coming from? My father?*

I started digging and wouldn't let it go. The first person I called was my mother's twin sister, Aunt Anita. She didn't want to vomit it all out at once. "Well you know your mother was messing with this man Gary." I asked my older brother, Darryl, "Who is Gary?" and he paused like, "Oh, shit."

I asked him, "Is he supposed to be my father?" He was like, "Sis I ain't gonna lie. You look just like that nigga."

13

Seeking My Missing Father

I want to tell all the women reading this that sometimes in life we have to move out of the way and release all expectations. We have the ability to walk around and have expectations of people because of other losses. We don't even know if they are capable of reaching these expectations, and eventually the expectations come back around and bite us in the ass.

Our parents are only human, with limitations just like us. My hope for the readers of my journey is that you can move out of the way and remove all expectations as you grow into the person you want to be. If you are an adult who grew up with an absent parent, my advice for you is to do your own search.

In life you have to play your part, because otherwise someone will likely point the finger back at you about what you didn't do. "You knew you had a father out there but you didn't go search for him." If you do meet your father, he might even say, "You didn't try to find me," while all the while you were expecting him to find you.

I try in my life to make myself responsible for getting what I need without exerting myself to the point of denying I need help. When it comes to wondering who your daddy is, do your own search rather than relying too heavily on what other people say and on an expectation that he will find you, or someone will just drop the knowledge of his existence, or lack thereof, on you.

Colorado, February 2009

All these people were walking around knowing the truth my whole life, but not me. There was no other information that any of my family would give me, or at least no information they were willing to give my worried pregnant self. "Just let it go Shirley."

That February I was lumbering around at our place in Colorado with my nine-month self. JR was on the road and I was alone. I called Aunt Anita. "I don't have nobody. JR is on the road." She didn't let me finish. "Of course, I'll come, but I have to be back in a week. You better hope that baby is on time." She hopped on a flight from Alabama and I went into labor.

We went straight to the hospital and it was a false alarm. They said that I wasn't dilated. "You have to wait until the contractions are three minutes apart." What did I know? *A Baby*

Story on TLC didn't prepare me for feeling anxious and I was certain that those first labor pains were just the beginning of what would feel much more painful. The doctors also didn't know that I was alone except for Aunt Anita, and the clock was ticking.

I told her, "I'm really nervous because I don't want to be here by myself." I googled "how to speed up labor and delivery." I took a tablespoon full of castor oil and the next day I started having contractions more frequently. That day, it was snowing so hard. My aunt had just gotten her driver's license, late in life, but she wanted it because my mom died without having hers.

Aunt Anita said, "Shirley, I'm scared. I can't drive to the hospital in this."

It was past dark, cold as hell and snowing like crazy. We have to do what we have to do. I drove myself to the hospital with Aunt Anita as the passenger.

At the hospital I was in labor for about eight hours. I would get up, walk up and down the hall, talk to Demi in my belly every time I got a contraction. "It's okay baby girl." Then I would go back to my room for the one minute of peace between contractions and stare at the TV hoping to see JR in Miami playing.

At one point, the nurse asked, "Do you want an epidural?" I didn't want any medicine. I wanted a natural birth without drugs. I went from walking and watching TV to another routine, in and out of the hot tub while eating popsicles. Then it was time. I was yelling to my aunt, "Hold my leg up!"

She said, "I don't know who the fuck you think you yelling at. Calm down." We weren't Mom and PopaAuntie, but the odd couple doing the best we could.

I started pushing and Demi came one, two, three, just like that, easy peasy. Aunt Nita cut the cord.

Later in the night, I was lying there feeding Demi her first milk and JR was on TV just grinning from ear to ear for the camera. "My baby Demi Smith was born tonight at Rose Medical Center." I was in the hospital two days and then my aunt had to split, but JR's mother, Ma, came to town. In my head I was like, *It's okay that he's not here. My man has a profession where he has to be absent. It's good, it's all good.* I soothed myself, *Shirley, y'all talked about this, you know there was a chance that he might not be there when you have the baby.* I stuffed the feelings under the rug and moved on.

It all went smoothly, but a cascade of other shit started interfering no matter how much I allowed myself to just accept things as they were. People were saying I was a gold digger because I had JR's baby and I'm from the hood. JR and I were babies ourselves, and I didn't want to add pressure on his career, so I did the best I could to ignore that negativity.

At the end of the day all any of us want is to be loved, even if we have to jeopardize things from our sense of self to get it. I didn't know that I was repeating something to get something. My mother was with a married man when I was conceived. She stayed quiet to not draw friction in his relationship, to not draw friction in her own family. I was doing that in some similar forms. "Shirley just be quiet, don't ruffle feathers." I didn't know my worth yet, so I pressed forward into spaces in my relationship, being quiet when I needed to speak up.

And don't you know, you put out one fire and another one blazes up? I'm telling you, 2009 was blow-by-blow, minute-by-minute, joys and pains.

14

Paternity Crossroads

When Demi was six months old, our little family of three was summoned away from our home in Colorado, back to New Jersey. JR was being charged with the wrongful death of his best friend, who died two years before in the car accident that changed his life. Other than the day he came to my house-warming party a month before his accident, I realized that I have only known the JR that walked away from the accident where his friend died. He survived with what seemed to only be external scratches, but there has always been something worn down in his eyes.

The court appearance was short, but full of cameras, reporters, and questions about JR's career. At the time he was averaging 15 points per game for the Denver Nuggets. He was to serve ninety days in jail in New Jersey, which got reduced to thirty days and community service. "Okay, baby, you can do this and I'm gonna be right here." I stayed in New Jersey visiting family so I could be nearby.

I was on Goldsmith back in my apartment with my brothers. A good place to return to for the month while Demi and I waited out JR's thirty days so we could go home to Colorado. One day, I was doing my cousin Shantel's hair, and you know how it is? If you are doing hair or getting your hair done, you shoot the breeze. She was like, "Shirley what is happening with JR and the court case?"

I basically wanted to change the subject. I just told her, "You can go online it's all there, the whole world knows." She pulled out the laptop and got to scrolling through. I looked down over her shoulder and saw the picture of all the cameras in the courtroom and me sitting there with Demi up on my shoulder. Shantel didn't stop there, she just kept clicking and clicking, the way the Internet will take you deeper and deeper.

I told her, "Maybe we can look up some ways to help JR out while he's in there." She stopped me.

"Shirley, did you know about this?" She had clicked to some gossip blog. It was a website that talked about this woman Myra who had a baby by JR.

I just dismissed it. "Girl that gossip shit is what he and I live with constantly. Don't pay too much attention." Shantel didn't say anything, just sat with the laptop and I kept braiding. We were quiet long enough for me to start thinking, *This shit better not be true.* This baby and my baby are the same age. That would mean he was messing with somebody at the same time that our child was conceived.

Shantel broke the silence. "If you want me to, cousin, I'll reach out and find out more. I'll reach out to her."

I shrugged it off and I was like, "Sure call her or email her or whatever. It is what it is."

I tried not to think about it, but the next day it was eating away at me, especially the timeline, things he and I were doing the month Demi was conceived, thinking about when he was on the road. I knew our relationship had to be about honesty, but then I got caught in thoughts of *How can I bring this to him when he is already going through such a hard time and just trying to get through these thirty days?* I reached out to get a message through for him to call me with his phone time and he did.

I was uneasy on the phone between us. "Demi is fine. Things are good with everybody." I wanted to do the right thing and not put more on his plate while he was in there. Then I started thinking, *Why do I have to hold this and go there by myself? If it's true, it's something he did, not me.*

He knew something was wrong. "Seem like you holdin back, babe. You okay, everything okay?"

I said, "I just have to ask you something. Shantel found some shit online that you might have a child the same age as Demi." It was quiet for a while.

He was like, "I heard something like that. I have to take a blood test." He didn't deny it, just went straight to the blood test solution. He was like, "If it's true, are you gonna leave me?" He started reasoning, "If you leave me, I understand, but please don't leave me."

I didn't know what to do. It was just another thing. Another thing.

On Sundays after church, everybody would go to Aunt Brenda's apartment, but that week, I was over there every day. I was looking for the next best thing to a mama. I would have Demi on my hip and would be over there cooking and cleaning and what have you. I found a picture of this baby on MySpace. Her name was Peyton. She was in a car seat and I was like, "Yes, that is his child." In that same way that my brother Darryl told me, "You look just like that nigga."

I printed it out and kept helping with the housework. Then, I just fell apart. I sat down with Demi on my lap on Aunt Brenda's bed, holding that photo and looking at it, and looking at Demi, letting the reality set in. Aunt Brenda came in and I told her everything. She didn't say anything. She just held me, and I soaked snot and tears into her shirt. Aunt Brenda took Demi in the front room and I lay down in the dark, no appetite, and curled up in the fetal position. I just wept and cried not even knowing at the time the full extent of the paternal-loss trauma that I was feeling.

Life had to move on, one foot in front of the other. I just told JR to get the test, and things moved on. Honestly, I cannot remember him telling me it was his. It was just what I already knew that became the reality. JR has another child the same age as Demi. I felt like I couldn't leave him while he was down and in jail dealing with the misery of a huge loss.

One of my generational curses is that my siblings and I all have different fathers. I wasn't bringing that along. I didn't want my child to have that even if it meant I didn't have another kid after Demi. But God gave me a purpose and put obstacles in my plan that I learned to turn into bonuses. In order to hold my values in place about no multiple-daddy drama, I had to shift my way of responding to those unexpected absurd surprises that so many of us experience. Peyton became my bonus daughter.

After JR served his thirty days, we went home to Denver, and life went on as normal. One weekend, while he was busy with training. I decided to go home to New Jersey to feed two birds with one hand. The plan was to visit my family in New Jersey, and JR's mother was having a hysterectomy and I knew I could be a big help. I was also thinking it would be a good time to do more research on this man who was my father, something that had started nagging at me again.

It started out as a short weekend for me and Demi that turned into a life change. JR and I were talking on the phone, doing the daily rundown of how was training, how is the baby, and he didn't skip a beat with what he had obviously rehearsed. "I don't think it's a good idea for you and Demi to come home."

There was a long-ass pause. I was like, *Am I hearing this right?* I was like, "You don't think it's a good idea for me and your daughter to come home?"

Mama Bear

Couples have different versions of how things go. In JR's version we had an argument. In my version, this news came out of the blue. I was stuck in New Jersey with only a weekend's worth of things for myself and Demi. *"JR?* We live there. All of my things are there at home." I had to tell my brothers, "We not just visiting. I'm moving back in. Me and my baby."

A few days later my belongings arrived via express shipment.

I had quit both of my jobs when I moved to Colorado, so I was going to need to figure myself out from ground zero. I was like, *Shirley, pick yourself up. Where did you leave off?* I did how I do, I kept it moving. I kept myself busy to avoid dealing with those intense emotions of neglect and abandonment. I put Demi in day care and went back to school part-time at Kean University in Union, New Jersey, while employed as a pre-K teacher in Newark. And I couldn't help it. I went on a mission to find my biological father. Something in me needed to know that I mattered.

Demi was a little version of me. I was a baby once. Did my daddy ever hold me? Did he ever look at me and sing to me the way JR did with Demi? Did I ever matter in that way?

My aunt was like, "Shirley, you don't even know him."

But I told her, "That's my father. I need to meet him especially since he's alive walking around out there. Maybe he wants to meet me too."

Wasn't nobody trying to just leave it alone. I was like a dog with a bone once I started looking, and it didn't take any time. And guess what? He lived near my apartment on Goldsmith

Avenue. I ended up back where I belonged, but with a child of my own on my hip who I wasn't trying to have be out here in this life with no family. I started focusing my energy that way so I wouldn't chicken out on meeting him. I told myself, *Demi has a grandfather. I need her to meet him.*

15

True Father

The other parent or the aunts and uncles in your life might be, "Hush, hush. What goes on in this house stays in this house." You might not get real answers from them because they are protecting themselves and think they are protecting you from pain, so you may run in circles going nowhere until you do your own research.

I didn't have a mold for me to healthily seek a husband. I was a woman who had an absent father. I had to do that work of finding the answers about my father or finding what answers I could. It is only recently that I can see how that effort to find my own answers about my dad has paid off.

Mama Bear

I was interviewing people and wrapping them up in my search. Aunt Kathy said she used to see Gary back in the day when I was a baby and would say, "You know that's your daughter."

I interrogated my mother's twin sister, Aunt Anita, on a regular basis. "Y'all used to roll together. Y'all probably switched men and everything. I know you know something." Finally, Aunt Anita found him on MySpace and told him, "Shirley has questions. I think you owe it to her to sit down and have a conversation," but nothing.

Most people's stories weren't getting me any closer to finding him until Sissy, the woman who had been my mother's best friend, told me he had a white van with red trim and that he was a janitor at a gym. One of my girlfriends and I would ride through the hood looking for him, and then Sissy saw Gary and told him I was trying to get in contact with him. She followed up with him and talked to him on the phone about me. Then I got a chance to talk to him. That's when I found out this man was married to the same woman since way before I was born. I was a love child.

I was kind when I spoke to him. I didn't want to scare him away. "Do you want to come over and meet me and your granddaughter?" I told him she was a year old. He agreed and came to my apartment on Goldsmith.

He took one look at me and was like, "Yeah, you mine, you mine." I was looking in the face of the male version of myself.

I didn't let myself have emotions while I heard everything

he had to say. Turns out he lived right around the corner from the apartment where I used to hold it down while my mother was on crack binges. Which was not far from my apartment on Goldsmith. So most of my childhood and my young adulthood, this man was in my neighborhood. We probably walked past his house a million times.

He said, "Oh, this is my grandbaby."

And my emotions started to leak out. I said, "That's not your granddaughter. You don't even know her. You don't even know me. I just want to know like what's up?"

He told me he was messing with my mother on the side during his marriage. I had an older brother by him and his wife. But not too many years earlier, my older brother got killed when he was twenty-one. He gave me his son's obituary. I was thinking, *So I am my father's only living child.*

He gave me his number and we talked, met up a few times, and he said, "I'm going to have a relationship with you. You are my child," but then I would call him, and he stopped picking up. No answer, no answer. One day I called him from somebody else's number, and he picked up. I was like, "Hey," and he told me I can't call his phone. He told me that he was now very involved in the church and the child from an extramarital affair would make life messy.

He disappeared off the face of the earth.

My mind was just blown. At first, I was thinking my aunt was right. I didn't need more heartache. Why did I go digging? For the life of me, I can't understand why he didn't even want a fucking relationship with me. I was confused. *Breh, you don't need me? You don't want a piece of who you are?*

Strange how the tables turn, and turn, and repeat if we aren't mindful of where we have already been in life and where we don't need to keep going.

I was walking around thinking I didn't matter, and it led me into the wrong arms. I was caught between the push and pull of self-worth and feeling unworthy.

After JR told me not to come home to Colorado, I found myself waiting to see if he was going to turn around and change his mind. After a while, friends started saying, "Shirley get back out there," so I did. I began seeing this one dude and fell right into a live-in relationship. It was abusive, one of those situations where you are in it, and have tangled the rhythm of your everyday life in it, so it is hard to see your way out.

I remember one Sunday morning, that summer of 2015, being on my knees beside the bathtub begging God that if he gave me an out and removed me from that toxic relationship I would not look back. I feel like and know in my heart that's why what happened a couple of weeks later happened. It was my desperate prayer to God.

On a Saturday afternoon in July, I was hosting a fish fry at the joint home I shared with my boyfriend. While I was doing my thing of entertaining guests, my cell phone just kept ringing and ringing with calls from JR. I figured he was wanting to talk to Demi. She was six years old and I had done my part well of making sure that there was open communication with her and her father. I would drop her at his parents' house for him to meet up with her there. You know, open lines of communication regardless of the situation between me and him. But something must have been wrong for him to be blowing up my phone.

I finally answered, "Hey, hold on," and I hollered, "Demi, your dad is on the phone." I gave her the phone and left them to their father-and-daughter time and went back to frying fish and hanging with family and my boyfriend. After a while Demi called out, "Mom, my dad wants to talk to you."

I ignored that request, because if he needed to do a switch-up with the visit schedule, there were mechanisms in place for that, and the way we kept things cool was to stay out of one-on-one conversations about schedules and meeting places for drop-off and pickup.

Then my phone rang again, and this time it was my brother. "Hey sis JR came by here asking me and Bo if he could have your hand in marriage."

"What? You kiddin me. *What in the hell?"*

I didn't know if I was flattered, pissed off or what, but I was in shock. I knew one thing, though. It made me nervous as hell to be at the house with my boyfriend and shit like that going down in the background. My boyfriend was the type to get angry with me if he even felt like shit wasn't right. I spent the rest of the fish fry trying to act as normal as possible.

My brothers just wanted what I wanted. They wanted to see me happy and they both knew JR had my heart, hell even my boyfriend knew. That cloud over our heads caused a lot of friction between us because anybody could see in my eyes that I truly wasn't ready to move on but I just did anyway.

When the company left that night, I hid in the bathroom to text my cousin Danica about the confusion of JR's request. I accidentally sent the text to my boyfriend, who was on the sofa watching TV.

I was like, "Oh shit, oh shit, oh shit." I locked the bathroom door and didn't want to come out. I turned on the shower to pretend like I was busy in the bathroom. He was in the living room going for it, cussing, *"What the fuck is this shit? What the fuck you take me for?"* I was scared out of my mind and kept listening to his footsteps knowing that if he left the living room, he was coming to confront me. He loved Demi, so I knew he would never do her any harm. I cut the shower water off because I heard him coming up the steps. I braced myself.

I started praying, "God help me find the right path." And he continued to pace around until eventually he wore himself out and fell asleep.

He went on the next day barely bringing it up. I played up the good girlfriend to keep his mind off of it. I got his phone and started deleting shit. In the meantime, when he was at work or I was on my way to work, I started hearing JR out about all his life transitions and how he wanted to give it another try if I was willing. He asked me one afternoon if I would pick him up from the airport. I had to do all kinds of sneaky business to pull it off. My story was, I was going to go have lunch with my cousin.

Demi was with Kawana, my best friend and her godmother, and I remember I was nervous like I was being watched. When I saw JR, something happened different from the other times of us half-looking at each other to exchange Demi. I could see in his face all the shifts he had talked about. We hugged and our connection was back, that friendship we had shared for eight years, that connection over our losses and how we had seen each other through those losses.

It sounds crazy y'all, but we went that afternoon to the courthouse to apply for a marriage certificate. We later picked Demi up from Kawana, and me and Demi never returned to the house I had shared with my boyfriend, a place that was once my home.

I was still moving through my daddy-abandonment, though. I thought I could fix the brokenness within the boyfriend and make him into good material. When that didn't work, I hoped things could work out with JR. I knew I didn't want my daughter to be fatherless. I also knew I didn't have a structure or mold of what a father is supposed to be like for a daughter.

Four years ago, right after JR and I got married, this man Gary reached out to me out of the blue. I asked JR to support me in meeting up with him again. When I saw him, I just flat-out asked, "What the hell happened?"

He turned back to his story about his life in the church. He didn't take any responsibility for his own actions.

I told him, "You're supposed to be a Christian and you can't even handle my existence? I want a relationship with my father that's all."

He just blamed it on the church.

So I settled. "You know what. It's cool," I told this man. "The ball is in your court." And he ain't picked that shit up, dribbled it, shot it in the hoop. He ain't done nothin.

JR was very supportive at this meeting. Afterward he just said, "Yo, babe, that's crazy." JR had also met Erics, the man I thought was my father who doesn't look anything like me. But when he met this man Gary, he said, "That shit is crazy. You look exactly like him."

I walked away from that situation of looking for my father all those years ago, saying to myself that I don't know how, but I don't plan to be part of this daddy drama repeating itself. At the end of the day, I was sad and disheartened, but proud of the effort I had made. I still had some question marks that are hard to walk around. But I have fewer of them now. Out of one hundred questions, now I only have twenty. I know what he looks like and how that is reflected in what I look like. I can now tell my children true, even if not flattering, stories about their real grandfather.

I am proud of myself that out of my thirty-six years of living, I sought the truth of my father in my twenty-fifth year. I did that, and I'm proud of that. Yes, in the beginning it hurt, but I took the necessary steps to have the truth in my life and that is healing for my mind and my body, and I will be able to offer my daughters that healed space in their family.

JR and I had found our way back to each other, and him back into the regular everyday life of Demi. I told myself, *Whatever I can do. I will do.* I was going to put the same effort I used to find my father into keeping my daughter's father in her life. With my efforts, I wanted to fill in a blank for me and for my daughter.

Today, as the mother of children whose father has an occupation where he has to be absent, it is very important for me to let them know that daddy is working. I don't want to repeat for them the lack of information that occurred in my childhood. I have been diligent in creating for my children a structure of fatherhood even if he is absent for work or absent because we might have something going on between us. I put that effort in and set the expectations for my actions so that my children have a daddy connection.

Dropping Jewels

Create Your Own Mold of a Good Father

A lot of us Black women grow up without fathers on the scene, which means we tend to work harder to keep our romantic relationships intact. We try to keep quiet and not voice our truths as a way to keep our partners, but we are really pushing ourselves down.

We don't want to live through the abandonment again. Who would? But our strategies don't serve us. We end up with our mold for a "good man" being based on an absent man. We try to seek relationships that fill in the broken mold rather than just scrapping the broken mold and building a sturdy, healthy one.

Imagine that you are walking around with a space in your head that is empty except for a question mark, and the feeling that without filling in that puzzle piece you will never be whole. Whatever the truth is, a man sitting in an easy chair or a man's name on a grave marker, you have to know it for yourself. You have to go find out for yourself in order to accept it. You will be able to say you saw it with your own eyes or heard the truth with your own ears. You can be proud of yourself for making the effort, for trying regardless of the outcome.

In therapy I came face-to-face with my daddy issues, how they impacted how I was feeling about myself and how I was looking for love. I wanted so much to be loved and accepted that I took on projects of love and fixed them up thinking that if I did, that person would love and appreciate me and never leave me.

I am saying to the women reading this book, that if the structure or the foundation isn't there the way you'd like it to be, you can still stop the generational curse, by helping your children have a daddy foundation if their father has to be absent. True that he has to deal with his relationship with his children, but don't be the parent who is telling the children what she thinks of their father.

Of course if contact is dangerous, that's a different story, but in the daily course of being separated for nonabusive reasons from their father, keep in mind that your children will feel loyal to you as their mother, and if you are mad at him, they will be mad at him. If you don't want anything to do with him, they won't want anything to do with him. Try separating your relationship with him from their relationship with him. Act in a way that helps him stay in contact with his children, even if you don't want a relationship with him.

So I work to keep my children's father in their life so that they have a foundation and mold for "father" and for male relationships, to the best of my ability. Here is some advice based on my own efforts.

On finding your paternal link:

- Put some posture in your back and know that whatever the truth is about your paternal link, it is not your fault. It's what you were born into or thrown into. But you don't have to walk around bitter doing nothing about it. Bitter leads to a lot of other avenues of negativity in your life.

- If you want to know, try to find out. Seek. Put the effort in. Regardless of the outcome. You will fill in the space in your head and heart that is a question mark. You will likely hurt over whatever you find out. But filling in that paternal puzzle piece or putting in the effort to try to the best of your ability will fulfill that empty space. This way you don't turn to needing the men of your romantic relationships to fulfill your daddy relationship. You still might end up with question marks, but you will at least know some truths.

- So take the journey and trust the process of seeking answers about the paternity link in your life. Putting in the effort regardless of the outcome is one of the only ways you can calm that part of your brain and be able to take up the reality of filling something in for your children.

Keep in mind what can happen if you don't think you matter:

- You have to convince yourself that you matter even if the men around you are reflecting something else. Otherwise you might seek love in an abusive relationship because you are not seeing your full worth.

- Fill in the empty space of "Do I matter?" with the love of your children, with family members, coworkers, church community, who always have positive things to say about you. If you have to, just hear their words about your worth until you begin to believe it yourself.

Now, on paternity of your own children and the baby-daddy drama we often accidentally pass down:

- When he calls, let the children speak to him whether you and their father are clicking or not. It is for your children, so that they don't have to feel the father-abandonment you felt.

- When it comes to an absent father, know that you can't force him to do anything he doesn't want to do. But you can leave an opening, an invitation, and a space for him to connect. For instance, you can let him know that you left a spot on the Christmas tree for the ornaments that he can make with the kids. You can't force him to take the bait of having a relationship with the kids, but you can leave the space open. Your kids will see that you did your part.

- Just do your part as their mother of making sure they have access to their father if that is safe.

- Lastly, be patient and keep in mind that his absence or reluctance to be with his children may be because of his own generational curses. I had to learn this for myself after I learned so many more things about my own pains.

PART VI

A Retreat to Reconnect My Womb to My Body

You know how I said, "Go to therapy!" I'm also saying go on retreat.

I learned everything about who I am now in this world and in my relationship with my children and their father by looking back at my daddy issues. But I feel like I broke the chain of abuse and found my self-love and the depth of love for the little girls that are my daughters by going on retreat. It's how I got down to my core wound with my mother and my feelings of being abandoned by her.

Retreat is so necessary, whether it's a half-day retreat, a one-night retreat, or a weeklong retreat if you can afford it. If not, get a relative or your best friend to watch the kids once a week and go to a free yoga class or take a free art class, or something online that you can do just to explore and nurture yourself.

It is through a retreat that I found and forgave my mother. I found and forgave myself. I found and reconnected with my own existence by taking a few days to let somebody else take care of me.

16

Finding Myself and Mom in Red Rock

When I take time and I look back at the tough moments from my childhood, I am looking from the perspective of a Black mother who has three girls to raise, a husband, and a household to run. I find myself checking to make sure each day that I have done everything right, and sometimes I have good days and some days I break down. When I feel that type of imbalance, I always try to go back to the core to see where that imbalance comes from. I feel like the tough moments in my childhood are the moments that shaped me into the woman I am today. The stress of being left alone to take care of my little brother, seeing my mom addicted to crack cocaine and not being the best version of herself. When I am with my three daughters and I consider my own childhood, I feel like my mother not only cheated her children, she cheated herself.

There is the person I know she was, very alive, very funny, such a comedian, but because of the stress in her life, she turned to drugs, and once she was addicted, she wasn't able to come into her whole self. I know the ways that all that life stress can grip you and hold you. I know how it was and still is inside my body, throwing things off balance and making it hard to find peace of mind in the midst of chaotic daily life.

One thing is for sure. We can't see our way to the healing by being inside the daily stress and chaos. It is imperative, and it is life-or-death, that you get away by design. This is when I learned that I had core wounds, that I was broken, that in order to be better I had to begin again.

You can't start over, but you have to begin again. If you really want a better life, to be hopeful, a better mother, a better wife, it starts with you. You have to let the old stuff die off and begin again. Go on a retreat, or to the top of a mountain. Get in touch with what is going on internally.

New Jersey to Sedona, December 2018
What's that Dottie Peoples song? "He may not come when you want him, but he'll be there right on time." There were ten years between dealing with my daddy-abandonment and finally getting away from everything and dealing with my core wounds with my mother.

A Retreat to Reconnect My Womb to My Body

The winter after hitting my mental wall and going to therapy and resurfacing all my daddy memories, I needed to get away to process it all. I looked at pictures of myself and I saw me, but I didn't see me. I didn't even look like myself. There were pictures of me taking Dakota to outpatient therapy, pictures of me giving Dakota a bath, pictures of me and Demi at soccer practice. The images are like looking at a ghost. I was doing, I was functioning, but I didn't see me. Then my brother's girlfriend gave birth to a preemie and I just wanted to be there for them, but it was a serious flashback. I needed to get far enough away from the stress to hear God, and to hear myself.

PopaAuntie was at the house so I was able to leave the kids in New Jersey. On December 28, I went to Sedona with my best friend, Kawana.

Dear Diary,
Day One Sedona Soul Adventure with Our
Guide Sequoia and My Best Friend Kawana:

We were in the red rocks today, climbing. The energy was powerful. We walked two and a half miles through the rocks. The views were phenomenal. We did a rock breaking exercise that was a physical release of years of pain, but then there was the writing exercise where I was able to write down to my core wound of feeling like I didn't matter. I have been carrying that in my body and on my back all of these years, but that changes today.

I do matter. I matter to me and I matter to my children. I truly feel like today is the new beginning of the rest of my life.

I will now reprogram and reprocess the new me. I will make myself a priority from now on. I don't need to be perfect, I am worthy of good things, of everything. I will start treating myself better than I have in the past.

Dear Diary,
Day Two after Sound and Breathing
Exercises with Penny:

My vibration was high, no words, but I will try to write my experience. Penny was so sweet and subtle. She explained that I would learn a breathing technique to take home with me to do once a week for eight weeks. I have no words for what I experienced. I just know besides the Holy Ghost it was one of the most powerful things I have ever had happen to me.

The breathing technique gave me a feeling in my body like it was tingling and about to explode. My hands felt swollen and I had no control, then my breathing shifted, and I put my hands on my pelvis, then my vagina area and I felt a healing in my cervix. Next, through my sound my ancestors were communicating with me.

Then, I saw my mother, she was on the red rocks. I saw her visually on the rocks and in the sky. She had angel's wings and she was so beautiful. She settled on Coffee Pot Mountain high in the rocks. My mom said, "I'm sorry, but you had to suffer to get the skills that you have." I then saw Jesus. His wings were huge from one side of the sky to the other and he was smiling at me.

Finally, I saw myself standing on the rocks, but it was my eight-year-old self.

I started calling out to Jesus. There was radiant light and butterflies. I reached out to my younger self and she was crying. We were holding each other, and she didn't want to let me go. I told her thank you and that I love her very much. I told her I am free and that my life has changed forever, that I rebirthed myself.

It was like when you see a baby and people be happy and know something is now different. I told her that's how people will see me, because I'm new, I'm different.

Freedom is an inside job.

I was able to say goodbye to the broken parts of my mother and my eight-year-old self and let the healing begin.

Dear Diary,

Day Three after Reconnecting My Womb
to My Heart & Soul, Transformation

In my last workshop, this sweet elder lady, Giah, showed me how to dance with my energy and release it back out. It felt good to channel energy and move it into breathing. She showed me a breathing technique that makes the brain sit on one wave and slow down the thinking: breathe in through my nose but breathe out while pushing the air from back behind my throat.

She then laid me on the table and performed NIS (neuro-logical integration system) on me, something I had no insight on. *She relinked my brain with the cells in different areas of my body to reconnect them all to work together. It's like hands-on healing, which she said is the best way to go. So I was slowly being healed in Jesus' name.*

Giah then took her jewel and as she dangled it, she said I have a stain in my heart from ten years ago, which is when I was twenty-four and pregnant with Demi. That pain I went through during that time made me feel that same core wound, like, I don't matter.

That was the time in my life when I also found out that JR had another child around the same time that Demi was conceived, the time I thought, I don't matter. *It was also around the time that I found my father only to realize he didn't want a connection with me*. I don't matter.

She then told me to climb backward in my mind to younger years and pinpoint what sticks out to me about not mattering. That was when I was eight years old and left with my brother when my mother went out on binges.

She told me to put myself in the scene. So I put myself at 24 South Grove Street in East Orange. I placed myself in the scene sitting on the couch in the apartment. She said put yourself in the scene and hug and hold your eight-year-old self and tell her, "It's okay, you are loved, and you do matter." The tears flowed down my face onto the table as I hugged my arms around my body.

She then asked me if there was a place where I would go sit and rest and be safe, what would that place be like. I said there would be sunflowers, water streams, waterfalls, birds, and rocks.

A Retreat to Reconnect My Womb to My Body

She guided me to go back, pick up, and carry my eight-year-old self and place her in that deep peaceful scene in my heart. I thanked my younger self, hugged her, and sat with her for a little while. I would take care of her forever; I would protect her forever.

Giah asked me what from that scene could serve as a re-minder of my eight-year-old self. I said, "A rock," because I sat her on a rock by a waterfall in my heart. She said when you leave out of here I want you to go find your rock.

Giah rubbed my head and hair, it was soothing. It was what I always wanted. And I realized that when I was younger, no one ever kissed my forehead or rubbed my hair like I do for my daughters. I touch them, I give them that comfort and that safe space that I never had. Then she picked me up from my back and kissed my forehead, and I lost it. I broke down.

The necessity of the tactile, the touch. Now I know how important that is. Not just to give it, but to receive it. Now, sometimes I'll tell my cousin, "Kimberly, can you just rub my hair?" and I'll lie on her lap and she'll just rub my hair.

It's not enough to just give, give, give love as a way to belong or to matter. We have to get that love and nurturing too. If we didn't ever have that from our mothers, we'd walk around thinking we don't need it. But we do.

That rock that I found to represent the safe loving space for my eight-year-old self is now in my office. Every time I look at it, I think about the love I have to maintain for myself and the nurturing I need and deserve from others.

I came back home and it was about to be the new year, two years after Dakota's birth.

New Jersey, January 2, 2019

It was Dakota's birthday, her second year of life. We kept it intimate. JR's brother Dimitrius was there. We decided to stay in New Jersey because we had family on both JR's side and my side. We weren't working and things were calm. Sedona had allowed me to appreciate who he was, who we were.

I felt anxious being away from Ohio, though, because none of the doctors there knew Dakota's story. I flew back a few times for her appointments. So much transition was happening. On January 13, I had a speaking engagement for the first time for Kota Bear and was anxious about that, but JR was right there with me cheering me on. Demi started at a new school and got into Girl Scouts and that was a lot of preteen drama. If I didn't have that transition of going to Sedona, I would have broken with the move, with speaking in public, with trying to help my daughter deal with the transitions of middle school. I mean a bitch would have broken, broken. But the time away on retreat, learning about myself, helped me come back ready to endure and open my heart in unimaginable ways.

Texas, April 2019

It was coming up on Peyton's tenth birthday. Some might call her a love child, but I have turned that around. She is my bonus child. She is not just the photo of a little girl in a car seat that broke my marriage; she is the little girl who with one look stole my heart. She is a little girl; it's not her fault. And I certainly planned to be a better woman than my own father's wife.

I had it embedded in my heart that I was going to take the girls out to see Peyton for her birthday. I had taken Demi out for Peyton's birthday once before, because I wanted Demi and Peyton to have the understanding of both families and embrace them. It was a milestone for both girls and for me.

JR and I were now married, Peyton's mother was now married. I felt there was a lot of growth among the families. Up to this point, Peyton was always having to fly to us.

I began to put a plan in place. We are members of Bluejack National, a residential golf community in Montgomery, Texas. It is the one with the golf course that is designed by Tiger Woods. The golf community was only an hour's drive from Peyton's parents, Myra and Rob. I said to JR, "Why don't we go to Bluejack in Texas, and go to visit Peyton for her birthday?" JR was super-uncomfortable, but agreed. We booked a stay for me, JR, our three girls, and JR's cousin Jalah, who wanted to come along for the adventure.

On our first day in town, I volunteered to help Myra decorate. We rented a vehicle and I went over to Myra's with all my girls and Jalah. JR hung back to play golf.

Myra said, "The party will be at the jumpy place but we are going to decorate the house the day before so when all is said and done folks can come back to the house and really party the way we do."

We had the music on. I felt accepted by her, and happy to be a part of something. I was happy that her husband, Rob, could see the good characteristics in me, see who his stepdaughter was with when she was away with her father.

I was like, "Let me see your wedding video." We all had such a fun and happy night.

Rob was so welcoming. "Let me run back to the store for y'all."

Peyton and Demi were running around playing on TikTok and with water guns. Myra and Rob's baby, Drew, and my babies, Denver and Dakota, were crawling age. It was happy baby chaos. "You got a pamper?" "Put this one in the highchair." It was like a mini family reunion.

It got really late and the girls fell asleep. Jalah and I went back to the golf course to JR.

The next morning was a beautiful sunny day, April 20; no need for jackets. On the drive to the bouncy world, JR and I got a little confused, because it was in the back of a shopping complex. I called Myra, who had the kids with her, to get better directions: "Girl, we going in circles. Help a sistah out." I was joking, trying to get rid of my scary anxious feeling. This was about to be for real. JR had never visited Peyton in her hometown. Soon there would be me, JR, Myra, Rob, JR's two girls who were the same age, and all of our children in one place. I can't imagine what JR was feeling. We got out of the car, and people who we knew and didn't know were talking to JR, excited to see a celebrity.

A Retreat to Reconnect My Womb to My Body

The kids got their shoes off for the bouncy world, and it started to flow. I asked Myra if she needed help with the cake. We kept it about Peyton. I was holding Peyton's younger brother, Drew, and JR got in the bouncy house and jumped with Peyton. It was a beautiful moment that I will never forget.

Myra asked if we wanted to come to the house. I knew from my own experiences of a girl wanting her father's attention that Peyton would love for her father to see where she lives, to see her room. I told JR, "Take me out of the equation. We definitely need to go. Your daughter is so excited to have you here."

Myra was so instrumental too. She asked Peyton, "Do you want to ride with D. Ma?" They called me Demi's Ma, D. Ma. Peyton was so excited. In the car she was in charge of showing us her world. It was like she was in *Willie Wonka and the Chocolate Factory*, "Turn here, now turn there."

You know the rest, how all the kid parties turn into adult parties. We were decorating Peyton's photo wall. There were drinks. The kids got in the pool. Myra and Rob put food on the grill. JR was holding a conversation with Myra's husband. We had the music on, taking pictures. It was both loud and harmonious.

Peyton came back with us to the golf course where we were staying. She got to stay a few days of that week with us. It was beautiful.

I offered Peyton what I wished I'd had with my dad. In some ways I was healing me through her. I didn't want her to have those shattered broken pieces like I had. That week I kept asking in my head, *Peyton, if I was you what would I want?* I would want my dad because Demi gets him all the time. I would want to be under one roof—siblings, mothers, fathers, and all.

This was like the opposite of the day I saw the photo of Peyton on social media and it broke my heart. We posted the pictures of our unique family online, and people were like, "The strength you had to have to do that." But when you take the adults out of the equation and let the next generation have what they need, love is what shines through, not who has cheated on who. All of the things that could come into play and derail things got pushed aside so we could focus on Peyton and the children. It was a weekend that no one will ever forget.

That weekend, I was thinking, *God willing this is not the only time we all will be able to get together, but what if.* We felt full and complete. There should be more of this in the world. I wish more women could get to an openhearted place like this so that all of our families could be healthier.

I was experiencing the benefit of having a mental break that sent me to Sedona, of coming out of that experience loving myself and having the capacity to love others the same way. God knew I needed my breaking point to happen in order for our connection with Peyton to happen. Whatever there is for me to do in order to prevent Peyton from being like me, the child from the other father, I am ready to do so that she knows she is loved.

17

Closing the Gap

I now had the tools to close the gaps in my life. Not only did I know myself, I knew my little girl self. I owed it to her to finish the journey of seeking self-love by investigating gaps in my memory. Just like with my search for my biological father, it wasn't about *if* I found any answers, it was about loving myself enough to take the responsibility to look for them. I was mothering myself by trying to fill in the blanks in my childhood life so that I could be healthier in my mind and body.

I thank God for the rhythm of life that Lynette gave me back in the day. It was an investment of her time, and of her love, and I was finally able to connect to being a kid. But there's the gap, though. She had rescued me when I was twelve. There was this big space of time between being eight, those days of Mama's binges, and being twelve and realizing Mama was on a long-term binge. I remember reading somewhere that the mind can hold on to events for a long time without even remembering them until one day, things are either really, really good or really, really bad in your life and you remember everything.

When I was twelve, I didn't remember the gap and that was okay. I was just enjoying my new life in my new community and life felt good.

It is only with writing this book and delving into the hard time I had with Dakota's birth that I remembered what happened in the gap. First it came like an epiphany, and then with the difficulty of full-blown memories. I'm glad I remembered, because it helps me understand even more deeply the things my body has held on to and the trauma in my body that came forward when I was giving birth to my daughters.

North Carolina, October 2019

After I started writing this book, I did a spiritual fast for three days and then decided to take the girls and go down South to North Carolina to visit my uncle Sidney, my mother's youngest brother. I thought I was going for one thing and in came a flood of epiphanies about my past. God is so strategic in that way.

PopaAuntie and Aunt Anita were there visiting Lynette and Kimberly, Keyera, and Kaylnn, who live in North Carolina. I realized that I held so much resentment toward Lynette for leaving me in New Jersey to live her own life in North Carolina.

A Retreat to Reconnect My Womb to My Body

I had placed all my abandonment from my mother on her since she was my guardian.

After visiting Uncle Sidney at the nursing home we were hanging out at Lynette's house and she was looking at me talking about how "Your mother was my favorite aunt." And PopaAuntie was talking about, "Your mother was my favorite sister. She helped me take care of my kids. She kept y'all so clean."

I was like, "Who are y'all talkin about? I think we are talking about two different people." I was so taken aback hearing them talk about her like she was a saint when I spent half of my life wondering where she was or handling her when she was high. The only reason we had any connection in the end of her life is because I checked out of my own college education to take care of her when she had cancer. I wanted to know her, she wanted to know me, but that didn't make up for the bad memories I held.

Before going back home to Jersey, I started my three-day fast. Hunger must have opened up a portal of memory, because I heard God say, "Call Aunt Anita," my mother's sister, and I heard, "Tell her what happened, that one of her old boyfriends used to molest you."

I told God, "No, I don't want to touch that." It was part of my memory that is the gap. I went into the living room where Lynette and PopaAuntie were spending another afternoon talking about the good ole days; and like it or not, my memories were regurgitated in words. All I could think was, *Oh shit! Oh shit!*

I was spinning around in the living room with PopaAuntie saying, "Shirley, don't kill yourself trying to remember all that."

I told her, "You don't understand. I need to see it. It helps it all, all of it makes sense." I think I was upsetting her, but I needed to say it all out loud to get it out of my body once and for all so I could heal. I told them, "I see the basement. I see the dirty mattress on the floor. I see some curtain hanging up with nails on it and my mother behind the curtain smoking on a crack pipe. I feel his penis on my butt." I was hollering, the way I couldn't scream and holler when I was eight.

It was upsetting everybody, but I needed to say it all, to get it out of my body. I told PopaAuntie, "I'm not going crazy, putting myself in a bad place, but you have to understand. It's all adding up." I hadn't explained to her my whole emotional and healing process of writing the book, just that I was writing the book. So she was wondering why I needed to do this to myself. I didn't let myself stop until I was exhausted.

Lynette stepped in and explained, "Shirley, the rest of the family didn't know where you was until I saw you in Irvington Center that day."

Her and PopaAuntie had never even seen my mother high. They told me that my mother ran away from the family, and they didn't know where I was from the age of like seven until the age of ten when Lynette started coming to pick me up once a week.

One thing for sure with our families and with our pain is we can't undo any of it. But we can get it all out in the open so nobody gets hurt because of being quiet or ignorant. We can go backward to go forward.

We talked and cried until two o'clock in the morning. I didn't realize that Lynette and PopaAuntie didn't know what happened to me because I didn't know what happened to me those years either. They only held the version of my mother that I never knew, and I held the version they never knew. They resented the way I talked about my mother and I resented the way they glorified her. It was healing for all of us and mended a longtime rift that I never really knew all the details of or reasons for.

My family of othermothers had supported me all my life, but there were some things, like looking back to face the pain, that nobody could do for me. They didn't know about so many of the pains I carried inside my body from childhood. They could ask questions but didn't know the right ones to ask because they didn't have all of the information. They could use intuition and rescue me without asking questions. They supported me, but until I gave myself permission to access and talk about the deep pains, no one had enough information to support me fully. My breakthrough was a game changer of healing for the women in my family.

18

Dakota's Voice

Speak up and speak out! Most of us grew up with everything on the hush-hush, and that meant we didn't have a voice.

Speak! Write it. Share it.

This is what I be telling women, that the value of us writing and speaking our truths is essential to our mental and emotional well-being. We have to allow ourselves to share the negative things and the positive things in life. It's all our voice and we deserve, as Black girls and women, to speak out when we need something and to be heard.

We have a tendency to hold our truths. We feel like no one hears us, and sometimes that's the very thing that keeps us from getting the medical attention we need in a world where our voices as Black women and girls aren't heard.

This became so clear to me recently when Dakota turned three years old and I found myself again standing in a hospital trying to get doctors and nurses to listen to me about my own child's needs.

I took Dakota back to Ohio for her first preemie visit as a three-year-old. Something wasn't right. The doctor wasn't able to pick up her hearing. They told me she needed to see an ENT (ear, nose, and throat) specialist and advised me to have a sleep study done on Dakota. They advised, "Mrs. Smith, you should go back to New Jersey and see someone closer to home."

February 2020, New Jersey

Even though I was from New Jersey, born and raised, and live there now, Dakota's life was saved at the hospital in Ohio. Her teams were there, and I wanted my child's team to be on the same alignment for her special needs.

I was reluctant, but I followed those orders. The sleep study was done at Robert Wood Johnson University Hospital in New Jersey. The results showed that Dakota had sleep apnea. Usually a child with sleep apnea will stop breathing once in the night, but Dakota stopped breathing thirty times in one hour.

The specialist said Dakota suffered from extreme sleep apnea and her adenoids were huge, which is why she suffered from so much constant mucus. Every day, Dakota's nose ran steadily and the mucus prevented her from being vocal. They told me she had to have her tonsils and adenoids removed to address the problem.

A Retreat to Reconnect My Womb to My Body

I scheduled the surgery for June 2020, and then, COVID-19 hit the world. I wasn't sure if the surgery was on or off with all of the precautions for the pandemic. To my surprise and relief, they bumped the surgery up to May and all was a go.

It wasn't clear if JR would be able to come home because he was in Los Angeles and travel wasn't advised. It had been almost exactly three years since I left the NICU and although this surgery wasn't life-threatening, it sent me back to the fears and panic of all of those surgeries where they didn't know if Dakota would live or not. The day came, and I was by myself. Los Angeles was on lockdown. JR couldn't get a flight out. I felt so alone.

Dakota was lying there in her little toddler-size blue gown with the opening in the back, tubes in her arms, and she was scared and so was I. *This is my baby.* Looking at her I see a perfect combination of my toddler face and JR's toddler face. She is us and everything we have been through and she is also her own feisty self who is supposed to be running around and making mischief.

The beeping noises had me watching the monitor. I yelled out every time there was a slight shift, "The numbers are down. What does that mean?" I was clearly panicky, pacing and feeling some of the trauma from a couple of years ago. I told myself, *Stay calm Shirley,* but I didn't want to leave her side. I prayed, prayed, prayed. There were the pressures of the past NICU experience, plus COVID was a fear lingering in the air. I whispered to Dakota even though she probably didn't know what I was talking about. "This is going to help you live the rest of your life to the best of your ability."

Thank God, the procedure was not long. I was in the waiting room reading my Bible. Then I spoke on the phone with my bishop, then ran out and got breakfast and as soon as I sat down, the doctor came out to talk with me and said, "Mrs. Smith, her adenoids were so huge. I've never seen them that large in a toddler, but she is going to be fine now." I went in to see her and she was pretty out of it. There was dry blood and drool, and I held her even though there were wires in her arm and hands.

As evening came and nurses were changing shifts, I settled my mind on another night in the hospital. That's when I got a big relief. JR texted, "I'm in the lobby."

There was only one parent allowed in the room at a time, but they let JR come up so we could do the tag-team exchange. We hugged and just held each other. We hadn't seen him in a few months because of COVID lockdown and all of those emotions flowed from my heart to his. I told him, "Okay, you spend your time with Kota." We swapped and I walked up and down the hall.

When visiting hours were over, he went back to the house and I stayed at the hospital. I felt more grounded that he was in town even though he had to get back to LA.

The next day, Dakota wasn't drinking her PediaSure and her tongue was sticking out of her mouth. I looked at her wondering if she was pushing her tongue out intentionally, but no.

Her tongue was swollen. I told the nurses to come and look at her. My baby's tongue was so big it was holding her lips apart. I told the nurses again that I really needed them to come and take a look. At that point I was still being polite the way we are taught to be polite in order to be heard, in order to keep people from thinking you are some loud Black woman. The nurse assured me, "We'll take another look soon but things are busy."

I sat tight for a minute or two, but that panic from the NICU days set in, all of those times that they brought us forms on end of life. That's when I paged the nurse again and this time stuck my head out in the hall not worrying about what I sounded like, just worrying about my child. I was a little louder, but still trying to keep it respectable. "Somebody needs to get in here. Look at her tongue. I need you to find the doctor. Somebody better call somebody, now." They just kept on rushing around. I was like, "I can't believe this shit."

I got a bit more demanding. I needed them to pay attention, but I didn't want to piss them off and then have them intentionally ignore me. "Excuse me! My daughter is out of it. She can barely breathe. She's stuffy sounding and nasally and her tongue is blocking her breathing. She is having an allergic reaction to something. Get in here and look at her tongue. Look at her damned tongue!" Unbelievable that they were still too busy.

I called JR. "I don't know what to do, her tongue is swelling up." He told me, "Calm down. Call the doctor again. The good thing is you are in the hospital already. She is there. You just have to get their attention." I went from demanding to yelling, "Somebody come in here and do something, now! Enough is enough!" I turned into that Black mother, that M-U-T-H-A!

Lo and behold the doctor came in, and looked at her mouth with a little flashlight, which wasn't necessary to see the way her tongue was swelling out of her mouth. "We are sorry Mrs. Smith. She must have had an allergic reaction. We are going to give her two doses of steroids to calm the swelling. This typically doesn't happen. . . ."

I was thinking, *Of course it typically doesn't happen, but it had to happen to my child.* They said maybe she was allergic to the rubber they had to put in her mouth to hold it open during the surgery. The swelling, and my nerves, calmed.

Every time the doctor came in Dakota freaked out. So I became the doctor and the nurse changing her diaper, feeding her, and monitoring her vitals. I told them just put the clean sheets there, her robe there, the diapers there. I did everything, but I was exhausted. I could not and did not sleep that night.

The staff were doing their job, but I am her mother and they couldn't verbally transcribe what she needed, but I could, so I did what I had to do. But I tell you what, by the second day, Dakota and I both wanted to get the hell out of that hospital and go home.

When they cleared her for discharge, JR came and picked us up. It was just like the day Dakota left the NICU all over again except she was old enough to make some noise or act up or do something to let folks know what wasn't going right. When

JR buckled her in the car seat, she knew we were leaving and going home. She totally calmed down and was happy looking out the window. You could tell she was glad to get some fresh air. I was so happy too, it was over.

When we got home, it wasn't long before JR had to fly back to LA, but when he did, me and my mommy helper Miss Pam took shifts nursing Dakota back to health. They said it would be two weeks, but Dakota is Dakota. She showed strong recovery signs after a week. Her voice box could project. There wasn't mucus or swelling in the way keeping her from being vocal. Her only side effect was her breath. Oh my God, it smelled horrible! She had a repeat sleep study done and it was 100 percent better.

I didn't even connect the dots until then that I was feeling tension about how Denver was two and had words that JR and I could understand, but we still couldn't make out anything my little Kota Bear was saying. It was not until those adenoids came out that it was clear that with some help she might be able to find her words.

A month later, I had a meeting at Dakota's school. They wanted to make sure that what they were doing for language at school was also being implemented at home. They made her a PECS (picture exchange communication system) board. The point was for her to communicate with us better, because things had gotten to the point that her frustration was just so high. She would be trying to tell us something, and we couldn't understand what she was saying, and we would be shoving stuff in her face. "You want this? You want that?" and she would just throw a fit at some point.

We purchased one of the same PECS boards that they had at school. The board had Velcro with all of these pictures. I've never seen anything like it.

One night, I couldn't understand what Dakota needed. She was crying and acting out in the high chair. I went and got the board and her book of pictures and I said, "What do you want Dakota? What do you want?"

She went through the book and picked out a picture of a kid taking a bath. The girl wanted to take a bath. I would have never known that all she wanted was to take a bath.

I gave her a hug. I also gave myself a hug, and I took her and her toys to the bathtub. She looked so sleepy and content and satisfied.

I had already created closure around my mother issues, or so I thought. I knelt down by the side of the tub, sponged bubbles onto my baby's back. There was her toothy grin, the way she looked at me, like she was seeing the sunrise. I saw that kind of love that makes peace with the spirit. I saw my mother's eyes. I can't even really give you words for what I was feeling in that moment. But I'm grateful to God for the healing.

I have since thought a lot about that day. Dakota had something to say, and I was there to listen. She had a voice even when she couldn't put her needs into words. That was something I didn't have, but she did the work and I did the work as her mother to hear her, and something in that moment was complete.

As fall sets in, Dakota is just months away from being four years old. To hear people tell me all the things she wouldn't be able to do, yet for me to see with my eyes that she is so independent, is a testament to her strength.

I have found a team in New Jersey to work with Dakota. After she was reevaluated, she started real school in a pre-K program. At first it was scary for her, then she started liking catching the bus. This little mama discovered her independence. She started telling us, "I am Dakota," "I catch the bus," "I go learn," "I play with friends."

One of my main rules for her teachers is to not treat her like she has a handicap. She is full in who she is. When I tell her what she is supposed to do, I expect the same from her as with my other girls. That has allowed her to blossom, and she is hungry to talk and communicate.

She has come so far from a little creature without skin, with me praying over her, to where she is now. She is a caterpillar who turned into one hell of a butterfly. Every night I anoint all of my girls' heads with oil at bedtime. For Dakota, I also anoint her throat, the place from which they said she would not speak.

She is a testament that you don't tell a Black woman, a Black baby girl, what she cannot do.

19

My Voice and My Mother's Voice

December 2020, New Jersey

Yesterday I had a spiritual meeting that was six hours long with two of my spiritual sisters. We do this periodically and just talk about our core wounds and what is really going on within our healing process.

My big sister had us do an exercise where we had to list characteristics of our maternal and paternal grandmother and grandfather, anything that we could remember of their lives or what they were like. I knew a couple of things about my maternal grandmother because PopaAuntie had shared with me that I was named after her, Shirley. I had a couple of bullets to write down about my maternal grandfather, again through my aunt's sharing. I didn't have anything to write down about my paternal grandfather, my father's father. I never even knew his name. I also didn't know anything about my father's mother. Not even so much as a clue of what she looked like.

I had to do the same list for my mother and father. For my father, I knew the things I'd gone and found out on my own, including the circumstances under which I was conceived. And then, I made a whole page of bullet points about my mom and the things that she went through. So many negatives for my mother. I was like, "Wow." I now know in my life why my mom had all of these negatives. That she was trying to use drugs and alcohol as coping mechanisms to mask the pain and run away from the things in her childhood. The same things I had been through.

The last part of my spiritual sister's exercise was to list characteristics for ourselves. It was crazy to see how generational curses drop throughout the bloodline without you even knowing it unless you write it down. Unless you see it or speak it out loud.

When we were done, I was obsessed with memories about the day I read my mother's journals two years after she passed away. It was before I even had kids of my own. It was a Saturday in 2008. A brisk fall day in September. I left work and went to Aunt Brenda's apartment to do what I had made myself too busy to do.

After Mom passed I busied myself with arrangements, moving, running from the reality of her death for two years.

Finally, I was ready to look through Mom's things, which were in a bag and a small box that I had under my bed in my apartment on Goldsmith. If I had known what was in that bag and box I would have peeled through them sooner, but I was young, and was dealing with my grief the best I could.

I had the box and little bag in Mom's big hobo bag with the colorful stripes. I walked down the steps to Aunt Brenda's one-bedroom apartment. We sat down in the living room. She had her black coffee with sugar, I had my coffee light and sweet. Aunt Brenda was good for cooking. She asked me, "You want anything to eat?" Aunt Brenda's was the place where I would go a year later to be consoled about JR fathering another child at the same time he fathered our first child, Demi.

"No ma'am. I'm good." I was nervous and just wanted to get to it, but with support. I thought that my mother's twin, Aunt Anita, would be the person to do this with, but she was back home in Alabama. We sat knee to knee on the sofa, put the bag at our feet, and took out the first thing, a green folder. Written on it in Mom's perfect sixth-grade penmanship: "Personal: Bertina Marie Harris, I Love You Today."

I looked at Aunt Brenda and asked, "My mom had a journal?"

She said, "Shirley, I don't know. Open it up and see what it is."

It was like she was leaving me a book she had written with a title and everything. The cover was tattered and worn with tape holding it together like she had been carrying it everywhere with her. I took my time just feeling and looking at the cover and Aunt Brenda was patient and rubbed my back, because the tears were already flowing.

I opened the cover and inside on the left side was her schedule for the day of everything she had to do from the time she woke up until ten p.m. each night in rehab. On the right side were yellow legal-pad pages with her same beautiful penmanship, and I had to blink to clear my vision and to right my mind so I could take it in.

I remember just going, "Wooo! Oh my God!" and giggling nervously at the impact. I remember Aunt Brenda saying, "Take your time, Shirley."

I read them all in one day. Slept at Aunt Brenda's and read until I was done. I remember that I felt complete. I remember that I felt like I understood my mother more after that. Of course I only understood her as much as I could. At the time I wasn't even a mother myself.

Something about the day with my spiritual sisters was leading me to go back to my mother's bag of belongings. After making my list of those generational curses, I felt like there was something I needed to understand all over again. I needed to see it all, hear my mom's words.

In my current house in New Jersey, I keep that same colorful striped bag in the top of my closet. I went to it as if it was the first day that I went to look at it at Aunt Brenda's house. It was late, around eleven p.m., and the children were asleep. As soon as I went to pour it all out on my bed, Demi came in like God's angel and lay down. Big eleven-year-old girl taller than me in her body and in some ways in her spirit. I went quietly about my business.

Mom's first journal entry:

April 7, 2005

My journal. I was suggested to start this journal by my counselor. I am in a spiritual treatment program/drug rehab. I've been going through some ups and downs here lately. I have attitudes, anger, resentments. I really don't know how to deal with life on life's terms. All I know and felt like was I wanted to get high and smoke. I basically wanted to take my will back because of the pain in my body. I just wanted to use so bad [in rehab]. I went through this for four days before it passed.

The sunny weather triggers me to want to use drugs. Rain depresses me. I'm early in recovery this time around and folks suggest that I stop being hard on myself. This task that I went through was real hard. I didn't like myself or like how I felt. I couldn't figure out what was going on and why I felt the way I did, but that was a part of the necessary process, I guess.

Exhausted.

Mom's last journal entry was six-months before she passed away. I didn't remember what it said from back in the day, and avoided it. I went rummaging through the other things in the bag.

There were her Alcoholics Anonymous chips and her AA notes.

There were all of the letters I sent her while she was in recovery, which were the echoes of the letters she'd sent me. It was like everything from our separate struggles as mother and daughter were coming together in that moment. The range of emotions I was feeling was like being on a roller coaster. One minute I was happy; one minute I was sad. One minute I was still and quiet; the next minute I had questions that somebody needed to hurry up and answer. My feelings were all over the place. My mother was so transparent in talking about her past, her hurt, her pain, her anger.

She talked about family, about incest, it was just so much coming from my own mother that I understood now from the place of being a mother. The worst feeling was similar to what I felt in the NICU. I could feel that tugging that a mother feels when her own child is in pain and she doesn't know what to do. This was as bad if not worse, because my mother was gone, and I couldn't do anything to soothe her.

The only thing left was to read her last journal entry:

September 4, 2005, Sunday
Went to the Love of Jesus, had a wonderful time.

I saw my mother in the choir, standing in her green suit singing. I stopped reading and just lay on the bed with Demi and wept. My daughter didn't even ask questions, just had the compassion to let me cry then get back to it. I read aloud.

A Retreat to Reconnect My Womb to My Body

Thank you Jesus for such a blessed day. The arrivals was Storm (Darryl), Shirley, Nita, Woody, Brenda, Kim, Kasandra, Lynette, Kimberly, Kalynn, Kiki, Lynette's friend, Danica, Walter, Sydney, Bugsy, Tisha, Pastor Barbara.

We sang our hearts off. The anointing was with us. This church was awesome. Sherry, Debra was there. I was happy to see them there. God I just want and need to tell you how grateful I am for you saving my life. You've given me so many chances. I'm truly grateful for who you are. You're God Almighty. Love you so much. I will forever love and be faithful to you. Please convict me of all things. You must, so I can live Christlike, like you.

These were the words of her heart, the light that I saw shining from her where she stood in the same outfit that I had her buried in, the green two-piece dress suit with gold trim and a jacket. She stood there singing that Donnie McClurkin song, proud and happy. This was her last journal entry. She was complete on that day, so many years ago when she sang her heart out in my new church home. She was complete. I was complete.

I now know the value of writing this book. Yes, it is my purpose, but it is also the blessing of being so vigilant to write in my journals. It is about documenting my life for my children, the first of which wasn't even a thought when I first read my mother's journals years ago. Today, she is beside me here on my bed as I read aloud, talk to myself, laugh, cry from the place of reading a mother's pains, thoughts, and wishes. All the while, I am a mother on this journey with my three daughters.

It is imperative that I continue to write my memoir, write my journey so that my daughters have my experience to feel what I feel reading my mother's journals.

I feel healed. I feel a sense of my mother's healing, like a couple of pounds are taken off of my shoulders because she left me with the answers to so many questions, so I won't have so many worries. I gained an extra dose of peace knowing that my mother did the work to experience freedom and true eternal healing.

My mother leaving her journals behind was not by coincidence. She did it for me, for my brothers, and sitting here with Demi, I know that she did it for her grandkids. Now it's my turn to do the very same so my daughters won't have to.

Today, I went back to my bulleted list of all of the negative things in my mom's life and added all of the things that brought her light to life: funny, loving, a strong will, with the desire to be a better person. All these characteristics I added to my own bulleted list. I have it in me to finish the work she started.

I don't know how my own end-days are going to be. I have to leave something behind for my daughters so that they will know what was going on with me, how I lived, how I felt, and that the struggle to bring them into this world was not one that I regret. I am dealing with my Black female life with the reality that I have been handed, but making the best of it so that my daughters don't end up stressed out, having trouble carrying their babies to full term, having so many mental struggles from childhood to overcome. My body, my heart, my mind, struggles the way that it does because like my mother said in her journals, I am doing the best I can.

Dropping Jewels

Reconnect to Heal from Loss

Two pieces of very important advice:

Acknowledge and heal from mother-loss, because that is the generational loss that gets birthed by mother after mother.

Reconnect with family by jumping over the barrier of family secrets.

Reconnecting with family is imperative to your growth and healing because without the truth you will be stuck in bondage. You will be stuck with assumptions and making shit up in your head for the remainder of your life sentence. I call it a life sentence because for me that is truly how it feels when you simply don't know and can't remember important details in your life because of trauma.

You will almost always feel stuck, trapped, useless, and alone because for some reason you cannot connect to your main source in life . . . which is *you* and the roots from which you sprouted. So by all means, yes please ask questions, yes dig deeper, yes look further to learn what you need to know so you can gain your own key to freedom.

Family secrets will break you if you don't make an attempt to unmask them. So before the shit hits the fan and causes more damage to your interior it is best that you begin to do your own heavy lifting of uncovering the truth. The feeling you get from simply doing your best effort brings forth a piece of gratitude that is hard to explain to anyone who has not even attempted to pave their own road.

Being open and honest with PopaAuntie and Lynette allowed to fall off of us all chains that we had no idea had shackled us. The release has been a beautiful sight to watch blossom within us all. Now that I know what that release feels like, I am committed to helping others get a taste of that freedom. How did Oprah used to say it on her show when she gave away gifts to the audience? *Everybody gets a . . .* Well that's me! You get a release, you get a release, and you get a release from all that is weighing you down woman. You deserve it.

At this point in my life I truly believe that transparency, release, and vulnerability have played major roles in getting me to this point where I can be so open and real with myself, my family, and now with you. It is time; in fact it has been time for you to dig a little deeper so you can come out on the other side. No it will not be easy, but it sure as hell will be worth it.

There is no deeper stress to the body than the stress of motherloss and grief. Yes, there is all of the other trauma, but my relationship with my mother was the biggest wide-open wound in my life that can now begin to heal and help me to be a better mother.

A Retreat to Reconnect My Womb to My Body

It took the birth of my firstborn angel and rock, Demi, it took almost losing Dakota, and it took the difficult pregnancy with Denver for me to lose myself and begin the long journey to figure out what happened to me as a child, why it happened, and how. Taking that journey has helped me to change for my children, so they will not carry on that loss. I had to do the work of healing not just my physical self, but my mental and spiritual self.

Having a premature baby is one of those life events that sends you back to your own birth. You have to go back to the beginning so that you can heal and be strong for that baby. You have to do the healing for yourself and have a starting point to become the mother you want to be. Not the model of a superwoman mother, but the real human being with wants and needs who is a mixture of the mother you want to be and the woman you are. It is so crucial to the point where if you are reading this book and don't have the funds to invest in your healing, set up an online fundraiser. Tell people to invest in you being a better person for yourself and your children. Invest in therapy, retreats, and your physical well-being. Ask them to sow into you. You owe it to yourself.

If you want to experience true freedom, you have to step out the box and do what you've never done to get what you've never had. You were born alone, you die alone; to be free and released and healed you have to do it for yourself. It starts with you.

If I have any more children, I am betting this healthier mind, body, and spirit of mine will help me to have a healthier pregnancy. I can't predict that, but I do know that my three daughters are benefiting from the example of watching their mother exhibit self-love and offer them all of her love, not just in my words but in my actions.

It is my biggest hope that no matter what happens from here, these drops of love and wisdom that are my life will have a positive effect on the health and well-being of all the women who read this book and the women who are their daughters. Because it is truly from my heart to yours.

Acknowledgments

Above all I would like to thank the Father, the Son, and Holy Spirit; without thee there is no me.

I want to say thank you to my husband, JR; I love and appreciate you. God loves and trust us so much that he gave us a miracle to care for and I am honored to be sharing this journey with you. I want to thank my brothers Storm and Bo. We all we got. I love y'all. Thank you to my bonus daughter, Peyton, for teaching me how to love unconditionally, without limits and stigmas. Thank you Aunt Frances, PopaAuntie, and Lynette for your sacrifice. I hope you are proud to see the fruit you produced in me. Thank you to my niece Heaven Lee' Aamari Glover, for showing me resilience, strength, and what it is like to experience Heaven on earth. To my dearest Danica I love you! Thank you for your gifts, your persistence, and your drive to please and overachieve. You have been with me, believed in me, and helped me from the start, and I have no doubt in my heart that you will be right here with me to the finish. God knew we would need one another . . . PERIOD. Thank you to my whole family. I love each and every one of you for the ways you have supported my journey. Special thanks to my best friend, Kawana, for always believing in me and just being there: "This is us."

I so appreciate and want to thank you, Nanny (Miss Pam). Without you being here, I would have never been able to grow and get myself together and heal properly without having your help with the girls. God placed you in my life at the perfect time so I could get this book done. You came into my life at a time when it was hard for me to trust anyone with my children. For showing and teaching me how to keep my heart right, I want to thank you, Bishop Barbara Glanton. The example you are to your flock is unmatchable.

I want to thank and acknowledge you, Zelda, for allowing me to be transparent and allowing me to heal throughout this process of sharing my life with you, and being my sister who gave me guidance and wisdom along the way. I feel like our relationship has grown and I've gained another family member throughout this process. I want to thank my agent, Rica, for believing in me and saying "Yes." Thank you for having lunch with me on that special day and believing in the story's potential. I would like to thank HarperCollins and the wonderful editors Amber and Sarah who dedicated their energy to this book.

Resources

Resources for Families with Preemies

My Kota Bear, Inc.: https://www.mykotabear.com/

Graham's Foundation: https://grahamsfoundation.org/

What to Expect: https://www.whattoexpect.com/first-year /support-for-parents-of-premature-babies.aspx

PreemieWorld: https://preemieworld.com/

PreemieCare Support Groups: https://www.preemiecare.org /supportgroups.htm

Resources for Postpartum Depression and Mental Health Support

Substance Abuse and Mental Health Services Administration National Helpline: https://www.samhsa.gov/find-help /national-helpline

Resources

Psychology Today: "Find a Therapist" Database: https://
www.psychologytoday.com/us/therapists

National Suicide Prevention Lifeline: 800-273-8255; https://
suicidepreventionlifeline.org/

Postpartum Support International: https://www.postpartum
.net/

References

Of particular interest in illuminating the crisis is Linda
Villarosa's piece, "Why America's Black Mothers and Babies
Are in a Life-or-Death Crisis." *New York Times*, April 11, 2018.
https://www.nytimes.com/2018/04/11/magazine/black-mothers
-babies-death-maternal-mortality.html.

Broomfield, Robyn. "African American Women and Postpartum
Depression." Master's thesis, The College at Brockport, State
University of New York, 2014. http://digitalcommons.brockport
.edu/edc_theses/163.

Lewis, Tené T., and Miriam E. Van Dyke. "Discrimination and
the Health of African Americans: The Potential Importance of
Intersectionalities." *Current Directions in Psychological Science* 27,
no. 3 (May 2018): 176–82. https://doi.org/10.1177/0963721418
770442.

Musgrave, Catherine F., Carol Easley Allen, and Gregory J.
Allen. "Spirituality and Health for Women of Color." *American*

References

Journal of Public Health 92, no. 4 (2002): 557–60. https://ajph
.aphapublications.org/doi/pdf/10.2105/AJPH.92.4.557.

Prather, Cynthia, et al. "Racism, African American Women, and
Their Sexual and Reproductive Health: A Review of Historical
and Contemporary Evidence and Implications for Health
Equity." *Health Equity* 2, no. 1 (2018). http://online.liebertpub
.com/doi/10.1089/heq.2017.0045.

Smith, Imari, et al. "Fighting at Birth: Eradicating the Black-
White Infant Mortality Gap." Samuel DuBois Cook Center on
Social Equity and Insight Center for Community Economic
Development, Duke University (March 2018). https://social
equity.duke.edu/wp-content/uploads/2019/12/Eradicating-Black
-Infant-Mortality-March-2018.pdf.

About the Author

SHIRLEY MARIE SMITH was born in Newark, New Jersey, on August 8, 1984. She is mother of four daughters and wife to two-time NBA Champion JR Smith. In 2017 her daughter Dakota was born at exactly twenty-two weeks, an event that brought out the depths of faith and strength in her marriage. Less than a year later, she suffered complications with the birth of her daughter Denver, who luckily was carried to full term. Post-partum depression set in times two and sent Shirley on a journey back to her childhood pains to heal and move forward. She travels and speaks on these experiences in order to educate and encourage parents of preemies and to offer guidance to women who have struggled with postpartum depression. She is CEO of My Kota Bear, a nonprofit whose mission is to bring support to NICU (neonatal intensive care unit) families. She is a seasoned public speaker, bringing awareness to the issues faced by families of preemies. She is also known for her workshops that inspire and empower women and girls.

About the Writer

Zelda Lockhart holds a PhD in Expressive Arts Therapies, an MA in literature, and a certificate in writing, directing, and editing from the New York Film Academy. Her latest books include the forthcoming HarperCollins title *Trinity*, a novel of a Black father, his son, and the granddaughter who set things up right again; *Diamond Doris: The True Story of the World's Most Notorious Jewel Thief,* by Doris Payne with Zelda Lockhart; and *The Soul of the Full-Length Manuscript: Turning Life's Wounds into the Gift of Literary Fiction, Memoir, or Poetry.* Lockhart is author of the novels *Fifth Born*, a Barnes & Noble Discovery selection and a Zora Neale Hurston / Richard Wright Award finalist; *Cold Running Creek*, a Black Caucus of the American Library Association Honor Fiction awardee; and *Fifth Born II: The Hundredth Turtle*, a 2011 Lambda Literary Award finalist. She is director at Her Story Garden Studios, inspiring Black women to self-define, heal, and liberate through the literary arts; and publisher at LaVenson Press, publishing for women and girls of color. Dr. Lockhart is an inspirational teacher, facilitator, and public speaker passionate about utilizing art to help individuals and organizations live and work authentically.